Neuroimaging - Neurobiology, Multimodal and Network Applications

Edited by Yongxia Zhou

Published in London, United Kingdom

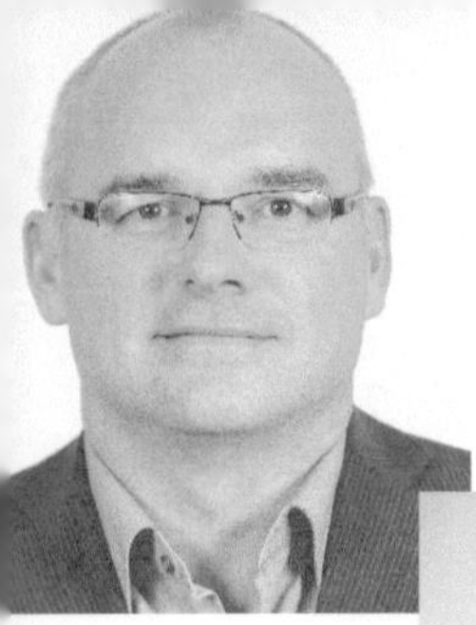
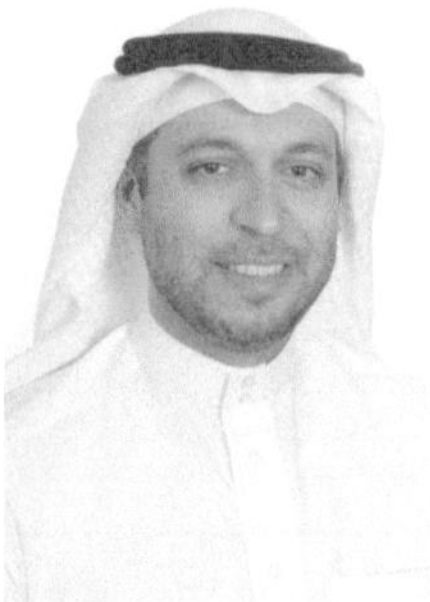
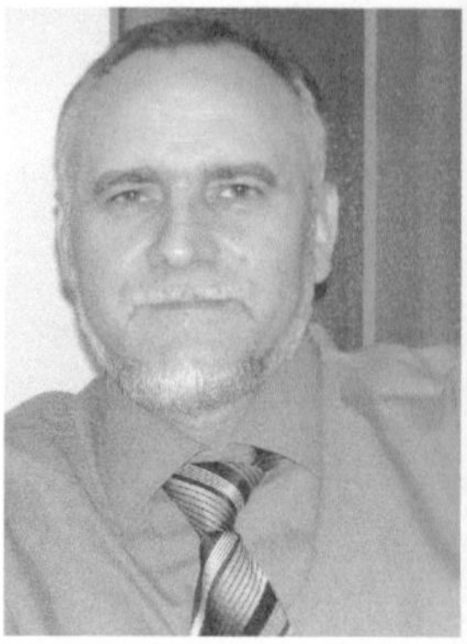
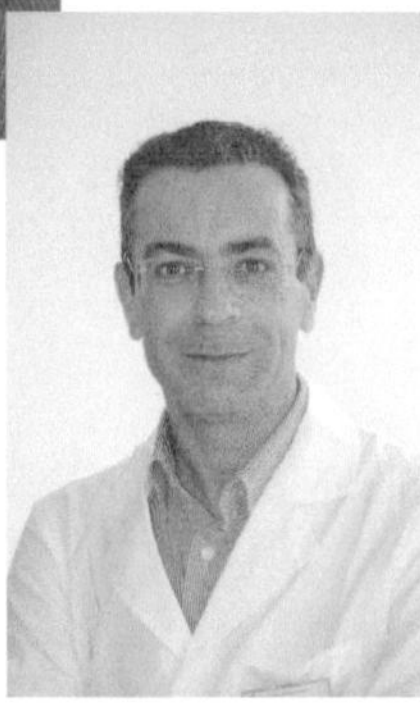
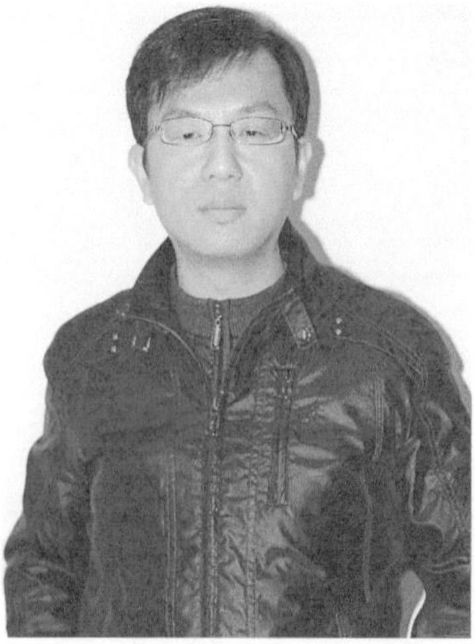
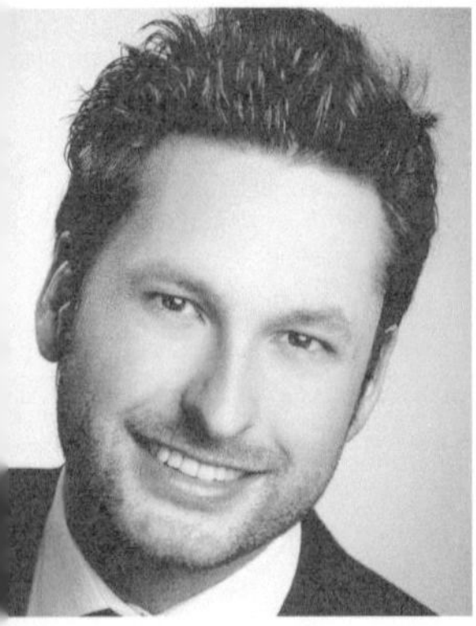
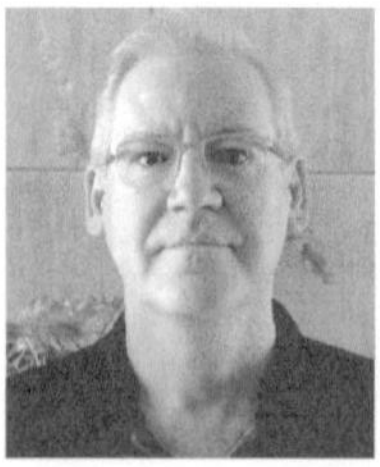

IntechOpen

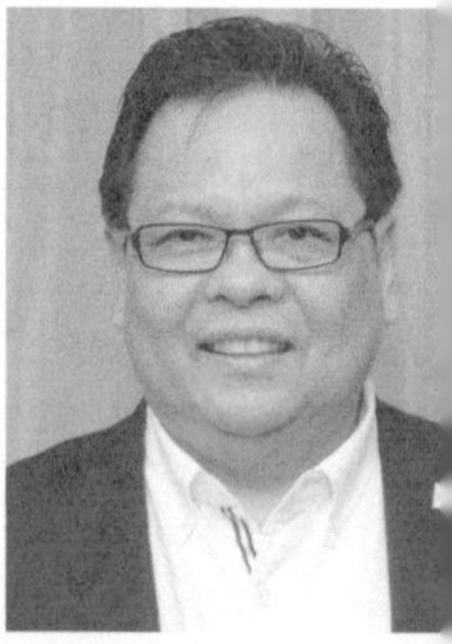
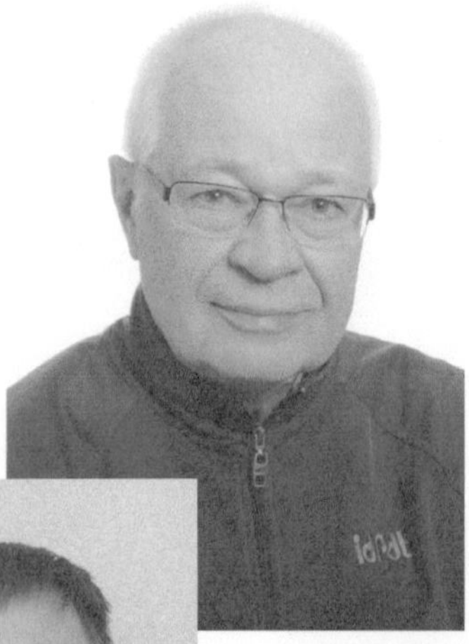
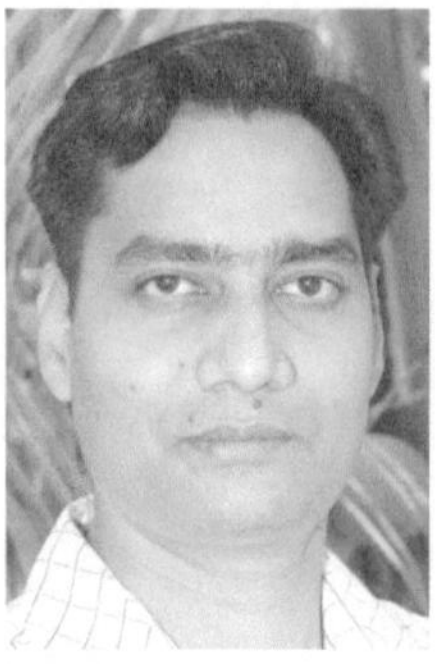
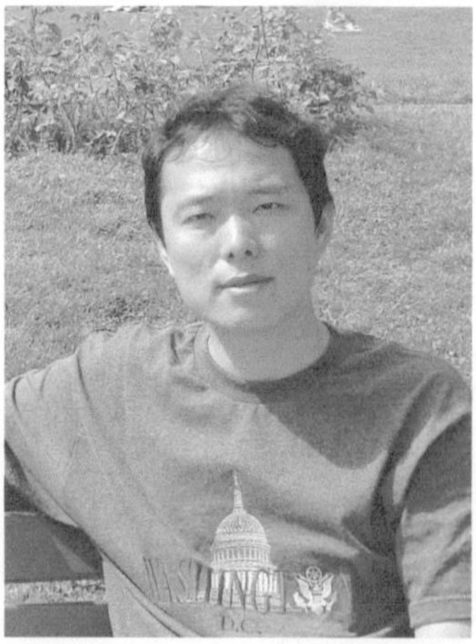
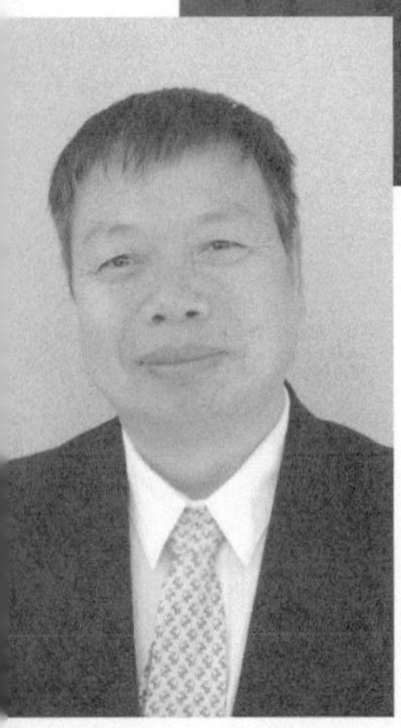
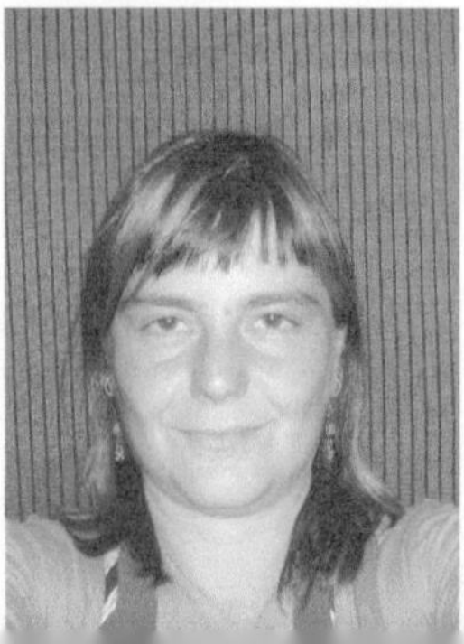

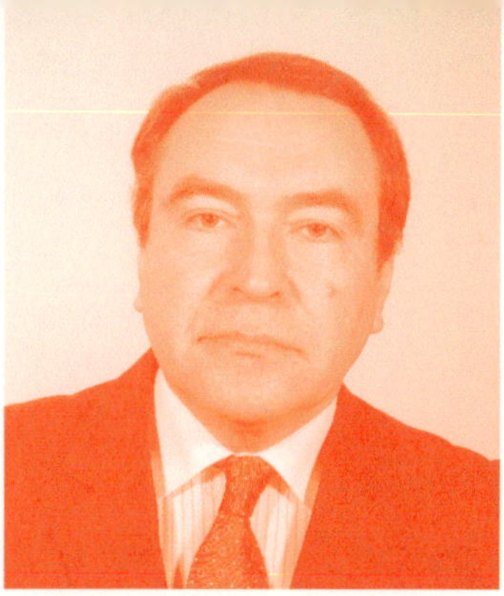
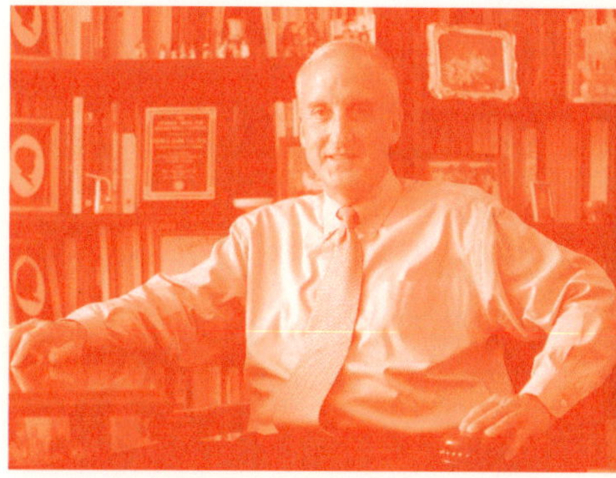
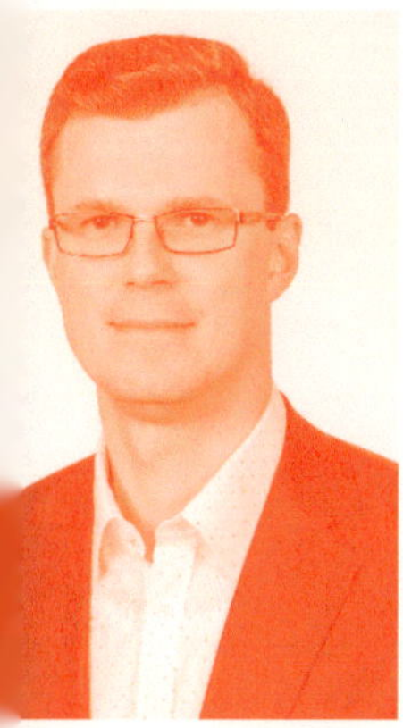
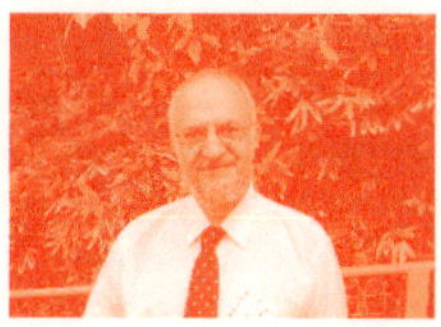
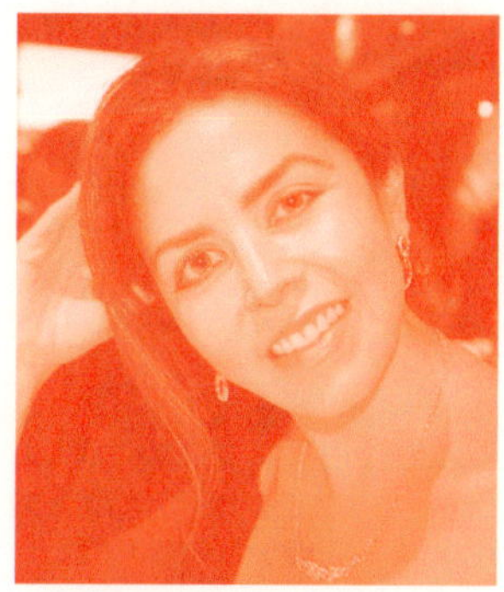

Supporting open minds since 2005

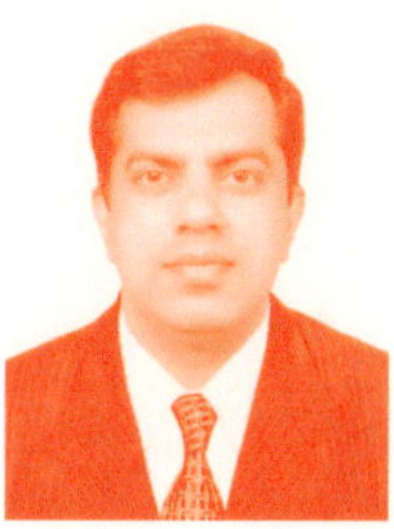
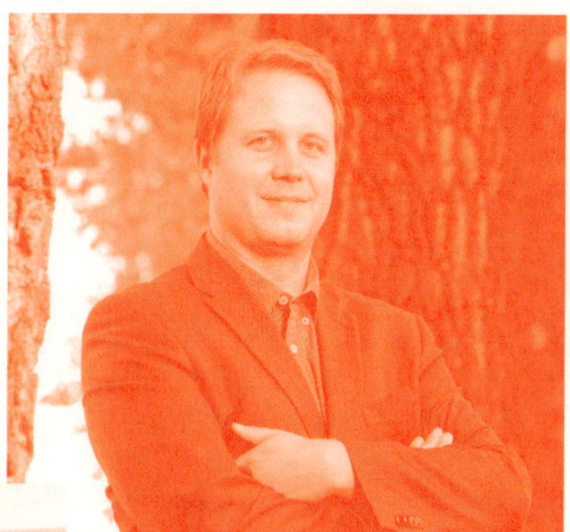
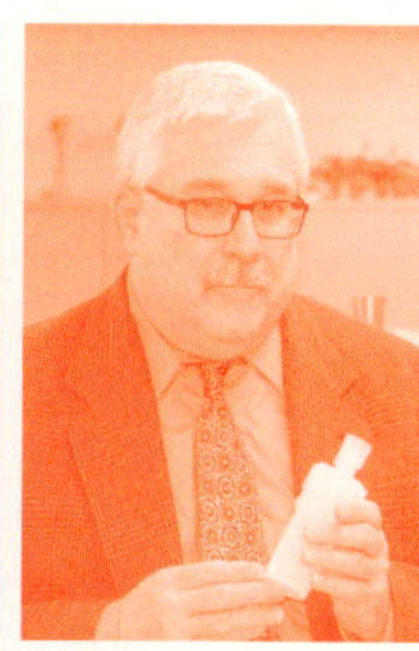
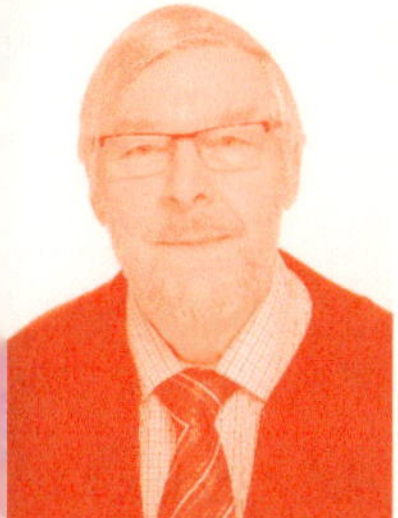
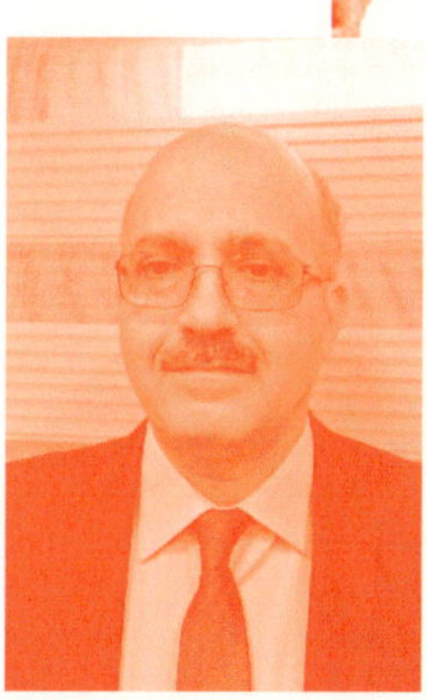
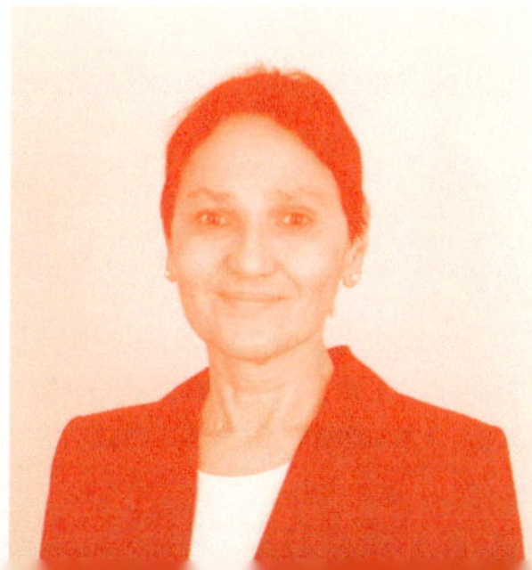
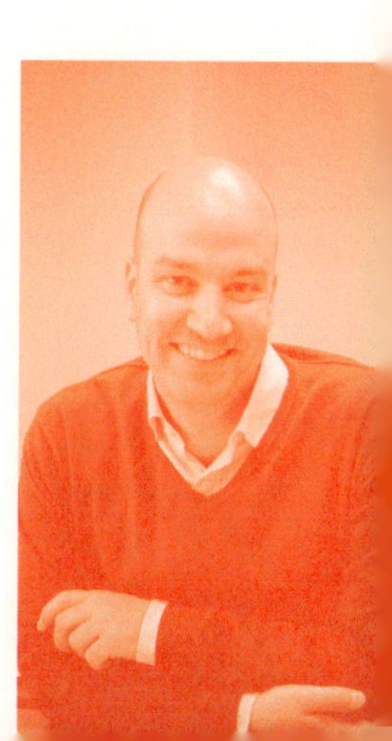

Neuroimaging - Neurobiology, Multimodal and Network Applications
http://dx.doi.org/10.5772/intechopen.83577
Edited by Yongxia Zhou

Contributors
Ali H Husseen Al-Nuaimi, Emmanuel Ifeachor, Emmanuel Jammeh, Lingfen Sun, Shaymaa S Al-Juboori, Thomas J. FitzGerald, Fran Laurie, Matthew Iandoli, Maryann Bishop-Jodoin, Richard Hanusik, Kathryn Karolczuk, Sandra Kessel, Fred Prior, Joel Saltz, Ashish Sharma, Michael Knopp, Mark Rosen, Ying Xiao, David Followill, Jeff Michalski, M. Giulia Cicchetti, Janaki Moni, Hitoshi Tsunashima, Keito Aibara, Agnieszka Reid, Jie Tao, Xiaoli Wang, Zhiping Zhang, Yudan Zhu, Jiwei Cheng, Guoyi Li, Frank Ho-Yin Lai, Maria Uscinska, Elaine Yan, Yu Yao, Shuzhang Zhang, Wei Wang

First published in London, United Kingdom, 2020 by IntechOpen
IntechOpen is the global imprint of INTECHOPEN LIMITED, registered in England and Wales, registration number: 11086078, 7th floor, 10 Lower Thames Street, London, EC3R 6AF, United Kingdom
Printed in Croatia

British Library Cataloguing-in-Publication Data
A catalogue record for this book is available from the British Library

Additional hard and PDF copies can be obtained from orders@intechopen.com

Neuroimaging - Neurobiology, Multimodal and Network Applications
Edited by Yongxia Zhou
p. cm.
Print ISBN 978-1-78984-430-6
Online ISBN 978-1-78984-431-3
eBook (PDF) ISBN 978-1-83881-077-1

For EU product safety concerns:
IN TECH d.o.o., Prolaz Marije Krucifikse Kozulić 3, 51000 Rijeka, Croatia, info@intechopen.com or visit our website at intechopen.com.

Meet the editor

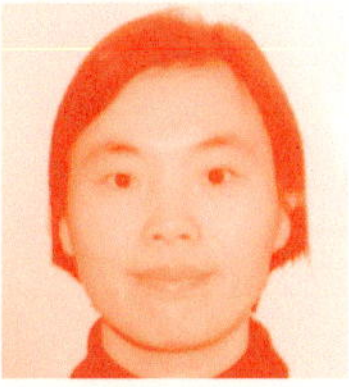

Yongxia Zhou obtained a PhD from the University of Southern California in Biomedical Imaging in 2004. Her main research interest is in radiology and neuroscience applications. She had been trained and worked as a medical imaging scientist at several prestigious institutes including Columbia University, University of Pennsylvania, and the National Institutes of Health (NIH). Her research focuses on multimodal neuroimaging integration including MRI/PET and EEG/MEG instrumentation that makes the best use of multiple modalities to help interpret underlying disease mechanisms. She has authored six monograph books, and edited several books for well-known publishers including IntechOpen and Nova Science. She has published more than 100 papers and presentations in many reputed international journals and conferences, and served as reviewer and editor for several well-known associations.

Contents

Preface

Neuroimaging is one of the main topics in radiology and neuroscience for probing normal brain physiology and disease alterations. In vivo brain neuroimaging with new technologies of multiple imaging modalities including MRI, PET, CT, and EEG/MEG has achieved great success with high spatial and temporal resolutions. Earlier identification of key pathological signatures of disease with advanced imaging techniques is critical for effective treatment and disease prevention. Revealing underlying pathophysiological mechanisms and utilization of ultra-fast and superior high-resolution imaging methodologies in large patient cohorts has broadened the neuroimaging field to the new horizon of precise and personal medicine. Multimodal neuroimaging metrics for clinical research such as functional and structural MRI, EEG activity, blood flow, and metabolism, together with the network management of nationwide clinical trial centers, are of vital importance and could play significant roles in improving disease diagnosis and treatment.

The first section of the book refers to the neurobiology of the central nervous system including neuroinflammation and fatigue perspectives. Chapter 1 “Targeting Neuroglial Sodium Channels in Neuroinflammatory Diseases” highlights the physiological and pathological roles of voltage-gated sodium channels (VGSCs) and their therapeutic implications for neuroinflammatory diseases. Neuroglial sodium channels such as microglial, astroglial, and oligodendroglial channels as well as their implications in brain diseases including multiple sclerosis, epilepsy, and Alzheimer’s disease are described in detail, respectively. The thorough review of the central role of glia in central nervous system health and disease could help further our understanding of the underlying disease physiology and molecular pathways, and therefore possibly facilitate novel therapeutic developments. Chapter 2 “Hypothalamic-Pituitary-Adrenal (HPA) Axis and Chronic Fatigue Syndrome in Older Adults: The Rehabilitation Perspectives” outlines the correlations between chronic fatigue symptoms (CSF) and hypothalamic–pituitary–adrenal (HPA) activity, the underlying physiological causes of CSF, and various affecting factors. After introducing the neuroimaging findings and clinical relationship between CFS and HPA, the chapter presents a randomized control trial examining the effectiveness of Activity Scheduling (AS) on individuals with CFS. The results found a positive effect of AS on improvements of activity participation in older adults with CFS, consistent with previous studies on depression. Revealing the biopsychosocial associations, this study provides insightful clues to the evaluation, management, and rehabilitation service for CFS.

The second section of the book covers the multimodal applications of neuroimaging including MRI, EEG, and NIRS. Chapter 3 “Neuroimaging Findings for Developmental Coordination Disorder (DCD) in Adults: Critical Evaluation and Future Directions” evaluates neuroimaging findings of DCD based on published literature. First, the chapter introduces definitions, prevalence, and symptoms of DCD. Then it presents detailed results including specific findings using each neuroimaging technique, providing insightful and perspective clues to the multimodal imaging evidence of DCD. These multiple imaging findings including functional MRI, diffusion-weighted MRI, transcranial magnetic stimulation (TMS), and functional transcranial Doppler ultrasound could provide a more comprehensive and complementary picture of the disease's functional abnormalities. Future directions including cutting-edge imaging methods and integration, longitudinal studies with more imaging metrics in addition to genetics are addressed accordingly with the hope of more groundbreaking discoveries in DCD research. Chapter 4 "Electroencephalogram-Based Biomarkers for Detection of Alzheimer's Disease" presents the application of electroencephalography (EEG) for Alzheimer's disease (AD) detection. This chapter illustrates research and development of EEG biomarkers that could detect abnormal AD brain activities based on quantitative analysis results of the temporal waves. Specific results including the slowing wave of the EEG and reduction in complexity are found in AD patients in comparison to controls. Similar to information-processing activities, three complexity measures extracted from the EEG frequency bands by TsEn, HFD, and LZC are significantly lower and remain consistently in AD, proving to be a robust and effective biomarker. Chapter 5 "Measurement and Evaluation of Brain Activity for Train Drivers Using Wearable NIRS" introduces near-infrared spectroscopy (NIRS) instrumentation for measuring brain activity during train driving tasks. It compares and assesses the blood oxygenation signal and oxygen saturation percentage change along the resting-task repetition paradigm and the real driving task. The brain activity of prior notice and increased attention could be reflected from the NIRS signal using the wavelet processing method. The results confirm that there exists difference in brain activity with and without prior notice.

The third section of the book introduces the Clinical Trials Network and imaging-related informatics. Chapter 6 "Imaging and Neuro-Oncology Clinical Trials of the National Clinical Trials Network (NCTN)" overviews and discusses many large data topics including clinical center imaging, radiation oncology, and data management of NCTN. It also evaluates the history, importance, and connections of imaging applications, neuro-oncology analyses portfolio, and cancer imaging archive. This informative and illustrative review chapter could serve as a good example in the field of imaging informatics' application in the era of large-size data mining for significant clinical and public applications.

Yongxia Zhou, Ph.D.
University of Southern California and Columbia University,
Los Angeles, California, USA

Section 1

Neurobiology

Chapter 1

Targeting Neuroglial Sodium Channels in Neuroinflammatory Diseases

Yu Yao, Xiaoli Wang, Shuzhang Zhang, Zhiping Zhang, Wei Wang, Yudan Zhu, Jiwei Cheng, Guoyi Li and Jie Tao

Abstract

The Hodgkin-Huxley model, at its 66th anniversary, remains a footing stone of neuroscience, which describes how the action potential (AP) is generated. As the core player of AP initiation, voltage-gated sodium channels (VGSCs) are always considered to be required for electrogenesis in excitable cells. Cells which are not traditionally been considered to be excitable, including glial cells, also express VGSCs in physiological as well as pathological conditions. The dysfunction of glial VGSCs is seemingly not related to abnormal excitation of neurons, but of importance in the astrogliosis and M1 polarization of microglia, which could induce refractory neuroinflammatory diseases, such as multiple sclerosis, stroke, epilepsy, and Alzheimer's and Parkinson's diseases. Therefore, in this chapter, we aim to describe the physiological and pathological roles of VGSCs contributing to the activity of glial cells and discuss whether VGSC subtypes could be used as a novel drug target, with an eye toward therapeutic implications for neuroinflammatory diseases.

Keywords: glial VGSCs, neuroinflammatory diseases, astrocytes, microglial cells, oligodendrocytes, gliosis

1. Introduction

So far, the pathogenesis of neuroinflammatory diseases, including multiple sclerosis (MS), epilepsy, Parkinson's disease (PD), Alzheimer's disease (AD), etc., is still unclear, of which therapeutic effects are not satisfactory, bringing great challenges to public health care. The pathological processes of these diseases are often accompanied by the production of neuroinflammation that cause a series of bad effects such as firing pro-inflammatory signaling pathways and even neuron pyroptosis, as well as cell death. The accumulated data show that neuroinflammation is characterized by the activation of glial cells and production of inflammatory mediators in the central nervous system (CNS) and peripheral nervous system (PNS) [1].

Activated glial cells, triggering neuroinflammation, include Schwann cells as well as satellite glial cells in PNS and microglia, astrocytes, and oligodendrocytes in CNS [2]. Glial cells are of importance for critical responses to neurological diseases and injuries, including active tissue remodeling, phagocytosis, etc. [3].

What's more, glial cells often acting as double-edged swords not only evoke the neuronal damage but also promote tissue repair [4]. Under pathological conditions, microglial cells, as one kind of resident immune cells in CNS [5], could secrete a large number of cellular inflammatory factors, increase oxidative stress of neurons, and induce apoptosis or pyroptosis of neurons. At the same time, M2 microglia secrete various neurotrophic factors and anti-inflammatory factors such as IL-4 and IL-3, which play a neuroprotective role in cerebral ischemia and hypoxia [6, 7].

Astrocytes are widely distributed in the nervous system, showing its function by providing nutrition and support to adjoining neurons [8]. Therefore, the excitability of neurons could be regulated by the neurotransmitters secreted from astrocytes. At the same time, it could synthesize and release a variety of immune factors to participate in the neuronal immune response. Oligodendrocytes are the unique neuroglial cells that form the myelin sheath, which is the key structure for neurons to propagate APs. CNS myelin hypoplasia or demyelinating changes are the pathogenic factors of neuroinflammatory diseases [9].

In the mid-twentieth century, after the discovery of AP, Hodgkin and Huxley, who firstly proposed the concept of ion channels, record sodium currents by using voltage clamp technology [10, 11]. Traditionally, glial cells were considered as non-excitatory cells, but with the development of research in this field, sodium channels have been found also to play crucial roles in physiological and pathological function of these cells [12, 13].

The activation of sodium channel is triggered by membrane depolarization, which produces transient sodium current and AP [14]. In neurons, sodium channels are composed of a single α-subunit, which forms ion-selective and voltage-sensitive pores, and one or two auxiliary β-subunits, which seems to affect channel gating and expression [15].

These channels drive electrical generation in neurons (Nav1.1, Nav1.2, Nav1.3, Nav1.6, Nav1.7, and Nav1.8), muscle cells (Nav1.4), and myocardial cells (Nav1.5). The typical role of Nav channels has been widely studied [16]. The dysfunction of sodium channels could result in neurological diseases, including neuropathic pain [17–19], peripheral neuropathy [20], epilepsy [21], and MS [22, 23].

However, the dysfunction of glial VGSCs is seemingly not related to abnormal excitation of neurons, but of importance in the astrogliosis and M1 polarization of microglia, which could induce refractory neuroinflammatory diseases. Glial sodium channels are closely related to phagocytosis, secretion of cytokines (IL-α, TNF-α), and migration. Then, glial cells are activated after tissue damage or disturbance, accompanied by morphological changes, enhanced migration, phagocytosis, secretion of inflammatory molecules (such as cytokines and nitric oxide), and antigen presentation [24].

Although glial cells do not produce AP under physiological conditions, they can show excitability through ion flux, especially in the form of $[Ca^{2+}]_i$ oscillation. Ca^{2+} kinetics is involved in microglial activation and regulation of many effector functions, including cell migration [25, 26] and release of chemokines/cytokines and nitric oxide [27].

The Na^+/Ca^{2+} exchanger (NCX) operates in a forward mode, transmits Na^+ ions down the concentration gradient to the cell, and then returns to output Ca^{2+}, or if the electrochemical gradient of Na^+ decreases or the cell depolarizes, the operation realizes the reverse mode by outputting Na^+ ions in exchange for Ca^{2+} [28]. Therefore, sodium channel activity has the ability to increase $[Ca^{2+}]_i$ through the reverse mode of NCX.

The research shows that Nav1.6 can generate continuous sodium current [29], drive the reverse operation of NCX, and generate the inlet. Ca^{2+} enters the cytoplasm. In this respect, like all eukaryotic cells, the intracellular free Ca^{2+} level is strictly regulated, which is crucial in the signal transduction pathway of microglia.

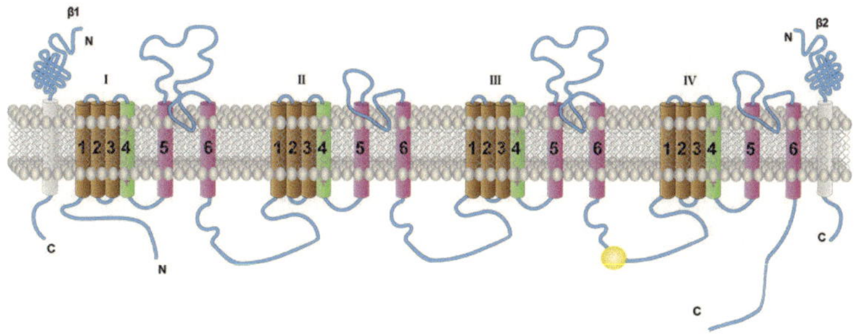

Figure 1.
Structure of Nav channels. Schematic representation of Nav channel subunits. The Nav channel α subunit is often illustrated together with auxiliary subunits β1 and β2; extracellular domains of the β subunits are shown as immunoglobulin-like folds (shown in blue), interacting with the extracellular loops of α subunits. Roman numerals indicate the domains of the α subunit; segments 5 and 6 (shown in purple) are considered as pore-lining segments, and S4 helices (green) make up the voltage sensors. The yellow circle in the intracellular loop of domains III and IV represents the inactivation gating ball, IFM motif.

Studies have shown that Nav1.1 and Nav1.6 were persistently reduced during epileptogenesis [30]. Under the MS pathological condition, the results showed that the removal of Nav1.5 from astrocytes could significantly worsen the clinical outcome of experimental autoimmune encephalomyelitis (EAE) [31] and the sodium channel Nav1.2 is expressed by scar and reactive astrocytes in plaque [32]. Studies have shown that under PD pathological conditions, Nav1.1 [33] in hippocampal astrocytes is significantly increased, and Nav1.6 is highly expressed in activated microglia [34].

There is a close relationship between the structure and the function of sodium channels (**Figure 1**). Therefore, in this chapter, we aim to describe the physiological and pathological roles of VGSCs contributing to the activity of glial cells and discuss whether VGSC subtypes could be used as a novel drug target, with an eye toward therapeutic implications for neuroinflammatory diseases.

2. Neuroglial sodium channels in multiple sclerosis

MS, a chronic inflammatory disease of the CNS, is characterized by demyelination, axonal injury, neuronal loss, and progressive inflammatory responses in the brain and spinal cord [35]. EAE is a classic model of MS, of which the pathological progress is very similar to MS. Under pathological conditions, glial cells (microglia, astrocytes, oligodendrocytes, glial stem cells) can act as regulators, effectors, and even targets of inflammatory response, not only causing tissue damage but also promoting tissue repair [4]. Glial cells are essential for critical responses to neurological diseases and injuries, including active tissue remodeling and phagocytosis [3]. Studies have shown that sodium channels are not only traditionally associated with the generation and transmission of neuronal APs, but also can be expressed in electrically inexcitable cell types including astrocytes [36, 37], oligodendrocyte precursor cells [38–40], Schwann cells [41], microglia [42, 43], and cancer cells [44–46]. The regulation of glial function by sodium channels is of special significance for the response of reactive glial to CNS diseases and insults [14].

2.1 Microglial sodium channels in multiple sclerosis

Microglial cells are the resident immune cells of the CNS. Under physiological conditions, microglial cells are usually highly branched cells with dynamic processes that can actively monitor the microenvironment of the CNS to protect nerve homeostasis [47]. However, under pathological conditions such as MS, microglia cells could be activated and recruited [48]. Microglial cells undergo significant immunophenotype and cellular and morphological plasticity in response to damage in the activation pathway [49]. The activation of microglial cells is related to the pathological conditions of the CNS. In addition, migration of microglial cells to damaged cells and pathogens plays an important role in microglial-mediated CNS injury and infection [50].

Microglial cells activated in EAE and MS are widely distributed and promote disease processes through a variety of mechanisms, including inducing effector T cell proliferation [51], production of pro-inflammatory cytokines [52], and phagocytosis of myelin. Moreover, studies have found that microglial cells activated in newly formed MS lesions are thought to be the main cell type that triggers the neuroinflammatory cascade after oligodendrocyte apoptosis [53]. Increased intracellular calcium and subsequent stimulation of the signaling cascade have been shown to be central events in the regulation of the function of activated microglial cells [54]. Studies by Matthew et al. have demonstrated that activation of microglial cells as well as macrophages is accompanied by upregulation of sodium channel Nav1.6 in EAE and MS [13]. In both the Nav1.6 blocker model and the Nav1.6 knockout model, the extent of inflammatory infiltration in EAE and the phagocytosis of activated microglia cells were effectively reduced, thus confirming that Nav1.6 was a key contributor to the activation and pathophysiological function of microglial cells [13, 55].

In another important pathological manifestation, migration of microglial cells to lesions of the CNS is a complex and highly coordinated process involving multiple intersecting cellular pathways such as membrane adhesion and retraction, cellular polarization, and receptors transducing external migratory signals [56]. One of the preliminary structural events in chemotaxis is the formation of membrane protrusions and high enrichment in the aggregated F-actin network [57]. In addition, actin-binding protein, calmodulin, and GTP-binding signaling protein Rac also are located at the protrusions [58–60]. The activity of MAP kinase and the reorganization of actin filament also play important roles in cell migration [61]. Importantly, Ca^{2+} signaling seems to have an effect on protrusions and movement [62], as intracellular Ca^{2+} levels can regulate cell migration, and the activity of a variety of migration-related effector molecules including Rac and MAP kinase is modulated by the levels of intracellular Ca^{2+} [63–65]. Studies support the contribution of the sodium channel Nav1.6 in a pathway that controls the extension of lamellipodial protrusion at the initial stage of cell migration [66, 67]. Sodium channels regulate Ca^{2+} transients in ATP-stimulated microglia and play a role in the activation of two key migrating proteins, Rac1 and ERK1/2 [48] (**Figure 2**).

In summary, Nav1.6 sodium channel is involved in the activation and functional regulation of microglia in EAE and MS and has potential value as a therapeutic target.

2.2 Astroglial sodium channels in multiple sclerosis

Astrocytes participate in ionic homeostasis, neuronal metabolic support, and the formation and maintenance of the blood–brain barrier in the normal CNS and react to form glial scars when injured [8]. With the deepening understanding of the importance of astrocytes in CNS pathology, it has been proven that astrocytes play a key immunoregulatory role in damaged CNS [68–70]. Though astrocytes have traditionally been considered to be electrically unexcitable, studies have

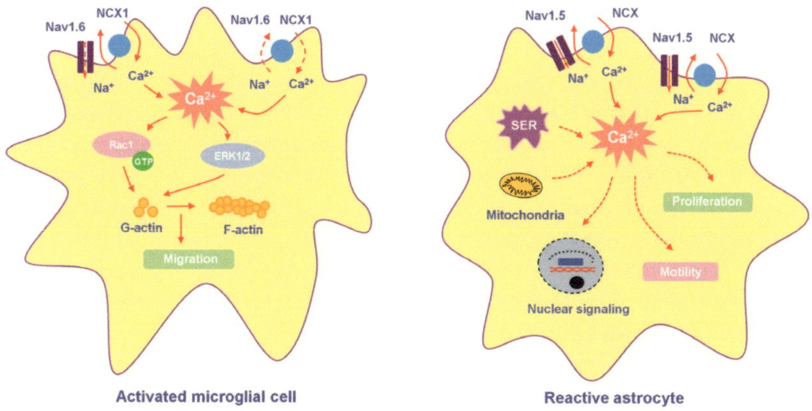

Figure 2.
Neuroglial Nav channels evoking Ca^{2+} signaling pathway. Schematic of putative cell signaling of Nav channel contribution to intracellular Ca^{2+} levels and downstream pathways. Depolarization of neuroglial membrane leads to activation of VGSCs (Nav) allowing influx of Na^+. Increased $[Na^+]_i$ causes reverse operation of NCX, which contribute to the level of Ca^{2+}. The Ca^{2+} signaling initiates downstream effects on neuroglial cell functions.

demonstrated that these cells express VGSCs [71, 72], including the subtype Nav1.5 [73, 74]. It is worth noting that the expression of astrocyte sodium channels in rodents is not a static process, but a dynamic process that changes with the age of astrocytes, exposure to extracellular factors, and damage [75, 76]. The voltage-gated sodium channel Nav1.5 is less expressed in astrocytes in non-pathological human brain but shows a strong upregulation of Nav1.5 in both acute and chronic MS lesions [71].

Different from excitable neurons, astrocytes exhibit their excitability by mainly in the form of $[Ca^{2+}]_i$ oscillations. Cytoplasmic Ca^{2+} levels in astrocytes come from multiple regions, including the endoplasmic reticulum [77], mitochondrial sodium-calcium exchange [78], and extracellular space [79]. The $[Ca^{2+}]_i$ flux of astrocytes not only regulates neuronal synaptic transmission, but is also important for many steady-state cell functions, including migration and proliferation, of astrocytes [78, 80, 81]. An important mechanism by which $[Ca^{2+}]_i$ is regulated in astrocytes is the reverse (Ca^{2+} import) activity of the NCX [82]. The positive pattern of NCX is to transport Na^+ to the cell and then return Ca^{2+} to the cell [28]. When the Na^+ electrochemical gradient is reduced or the cell depolarizes, NCX outputs Na + in exchange for Ca^{2+} by running in reverse mode [82, 83]. Therefore, sodium channel activity has the ability to increase $[Ca^{2+}]_i$ through the reverse pattern of NCX [82]. Interestingly, mechanical strain injury increases intracellular Na^+, causing NCX to operate in a reverse mode in cortical astrocytes, increasing the level of $[Ca^{2+}]_i$ [84].

Recent studies have shown that Nav1.5 plays an important role in in vitro models of glial injury by triggering the reverse mode operation of the NCX [71, 74]. Laura et al. confirmed that in the conditional knockout Nav1.5 model in astrocytes, the absence of Nav1.5 leads to a significant deterioration in the clinical outcome of EAE and an increase in inflammatory infiltration [31]. While the previous studies of MS in vivo models have shown that a variety of voltage-gated sodium channel blockers, including phenytoin [85], lamotrigine [86], carbamazepine [85], and safinamide and flecainide (Nav1.5 blocker) [87], could improve the clinical status and axonal damage, this suggests that Nav1.5 and NCX may be potential targets for the treatment of MS by acting on $[Ca^{2+}]_i$ to regulate astrocyte proliferation (**Figure 2**).

2.3 Oligodentroglial sodium channels in multiple sclerosis

During the development of CNS, oligodendrocytes (NG2 cells) originating in different regions of the brain migrate to their destinations to participate in the development [88, 89]. The directed migration of these glial progenitor cells is critical not only for the formation of myelin in the developing brain, but also for the repair of myelin after injury [90, 91]. Although NG2 cells express VGSC, they only trigger transient depolarization and fail to produce typical APs [92, 93]. Studies have found that intracellular Na^+ and Ca^{2+} levels, membrane depolarization, and migration ability of NG2 cells increased after the application of GABA [93]. While in the siRNA knockdown or blocking sodium channel model, the increasing tendency of $[Na^+]_i$ and $[Ca^{2+}]_i$ was significantly reduced, and cell migration was suppressed [93]. Moreover, a similar reduced $[Ca^{2+}]_i$ and decreased cell migration were also shown in the NCX siRNA knockdown and blocker models [93].

In general, GABA induced the depolarization of the NG2 cells and activated the sustained Na^+ current, which reverted the activity of type I Na^+/Ca^{2+} exchangers (NCX1) to evoke the increase of $[Ca^{2+}]_i$ [93]. Significantly, further evidence suggests that this unique pathway is associated with NG2 cell migration [93, 94]. Therefore, the important role of non-inactivated Na^+ channels and NCXs in the development and function of NG2 glial cells in the brain suggests its potential values in myelin repair.

3. Neuroglial sodium channels in epilepsy

Epilepsy is a kind of chronic brain dysfunction syndrome caused by abnormal firing of neurons, which has been listed as one of the five major neuropsychiatric diseases by the World Health Organization (WHO). At present, the number of epilepsy patients has reached 65 million worldwide [95], and especially the developing countries account for four fifths of this number [96], bringing serious economic burden to the patients' families and their country.

The previous studies on epilepsy were focused on clarifying the mechanisms of neuron dysfunction as well as neural network. In recent years, the researches on glial cells regulating neuron activity have surfaced with increasing frequency, which provide sufficient evidence for the involvement of glial cells in inducing epilepsy [95]. Glial hyperplasia is an important hallmark in the course of epilepsy; it refers to a spectrum of physicochemical and physiological changes in glial cells, particularly in astrocytes and microglia. The activation of astrocytes after epileptic seizure may be beneficial to the recovery of extracellular homeostasis [97]. However, more and more evidence proved that reactive glial cells could induce neuroinflammation by releasing the cytokines, chemokines, and other molecules, which is likely to cause neuron death, tissue damage, and microglial hyperplasia [98]. Unrestrained reactive gliosis might also cause hippocampal sclerosis, disturbing the normal physiological regulation function and promoting the epileptic seizure [99].

Glial cells express several types of ion channels. The Cl^-, K^+, H^+, and Ca^{2+} channels have been found to express in microglia, and the Kir [100] and Na^+ channels are highly expressed in astrocytes, which have been implicated in multiple functions of these cells [101]. These channels of different subtypes can be involved in regulating the membrane potential, migration, phagocytosis, intracellular ion concentration, and secretion of various cytokines and chemokines in glial cells [102].

Genetic studies have shown that the mutations associated with epilepsy mainly occur in genes encoding sodium channels [103]. VGSCs are a class of voltage-dependent ion channels that are highly expressed not only in excitable cells [104], but also in non-excited cells, such as astrocytes, oligodendrocytes, microglial cells, etc. [105]. Recently, it has been found that sodium channel plays an important role in the activation of glial cells and may become a new target for antiepileptic drugs.

3.1 Astroglial sodium channels in epilepsy

Neuronal excitability is closely related to the movement of sodium or potassium across the extracellular space (ECS). Because of the narrow volume of this space, the extremely small fluxes could also evoke significant changes in anion concentration [95]. Normally, a single AP can increase the extracellular K^+ concentration by nearly 1 mM. However, at the epileptic seizure period, the continuous neuron firing could raise the potassium concentration from the normal level ~3 mM to 12 mM [106]. In normal brain, neurons rapidly regulate K^+ concentration to 3 mM through Na^+/K^+ ATPase, and Na^+ activates Na^+/K^+ ATPase activity through VGSCs in astrocytes, providing an important feedback pathway for regulating K^+ level in extracellular space and maintaining stability of the central nervous system [106].

Thus far more and more reports have mentioned that sodium channel subtypes are widely distributed in most CNS glial cells [72, 107], including the TTX-S sodium channel Nav1.3 and Nav1.6 as well as TTX-R sodium channel Nav1.5 [14]. In the post-status epilepticus (SE) model induced by kainic acid (KA) intrahippocampal injection, the expression of Nav1.6 in ipsilateral hippocampal peaked at 21 days in astrocytes. On the contrary, there was no change in the expression of astrocyte Nav1.6 in the PTZ-induced epileptic seizure models, indicating that astrocyte Nav1.6 played a crucial role in promoting the epileptic process, but not in seizure period [108].

It is known to all that the voltage-gated sodium channel is composed of one α subunit and two auxiliary β subunits [109]. Co-expressed with α subunits, β subunits could significantly increase the current density of sodium channels, which is partly due to the enhancement effects of β subunits on the expression of sodium channels [110]. In the chronic epilepsy model induced by electrical stimulation, sodium channel $\beta1$ subunits are colocalized with the reactive astrocytes, and the number of positive cells significantly enhanced a week after SE, so it is speculated that the $\beta1$ subunits could interact with extracellular matrix, promoting the network of intercellular synapses in the process of epilepsy [111].

3.2 Microglial sodium channels in epilepsy

Microglia, as resident cells in the CNS, provide continuous immunosurveillance for the brain as well as the spinal cord [47]. When the body is invaded by exogenous substances, microglial cells respond to ATP or other cell signals, activated rapidly so as to provide immune defense. However, microglia cells can produce inflammatory factors in pathological conditions, causing damage to the body [49]. Microglial cells always express a large number of ion channels and surface receptors, which can induce relevant signaling pathways to convert extracellular changes into intracellular responses.

VGSCs are also distributed in microglial cells. Studies have shown that microglia not only express the TTX sensitivity sodium channels (Nav1.6 [13] and Nav1.1 [14]), but also express the Nav1.5 [14] (a TTX-resistant sodium channel) [14]. The blockade sodium channels of TTX and phenytoin could significantly weaken a variety of functions of activated microglia cells [12], such as the release of inflammatory cytokines [12, 102]. After a week of spontaneous epilepsy induced by electrical stimulation, the sodium channel subtypes were found to be highly expressed in microglial cells [112]. The Nax channel encoded by the SCN7A gene was observed to be significantly increased during the onset and development of epilepsy, and especially the high expression of Nax was detected in hippocampal sclerosis tissues from drug-resistant patients [113].

Ocasepine, as a clinical drug that targeted on VGSCs, is often used to suppress the epileptic seizure clinically. This drug has been found that it could significantly reduce the number of activated astrocytes as well as microglial cells in the hippocampus CA1 region in cerebral ischemia model, which also reduce the neuron death in the hippocampus caused by ischemia [14]. It implies that sodium channels are involved in microglia activation, which could also promote the progression of neuroinflammatory disease, such as epileptogenesis.

4. Neuroglial sodium channels in neurodegenerative diseases

4.1 Neuroglial sodium channels in Alzheimer's disease

AD is the most common progressive neurodegenerative disease, which is characterized by dystrophic neurites, neurofibrillary tangles, brain atrophy amyloid plaques, and loss of neurons and synapses [114]. In addition, AD is the cause of dementia and seriously affects the quality of life of the elderly [115]. Accumulated data show that the genetic mechanism of AD is mainly the accumulation of Aβ peptides and their aggregation in and deposition in amyloid plaques [116, 117]. The human genetics of familial AD also suggested that excessive production of amyloidogenic Aβ is a cause of early-onset AD; mutations in amyloid precursor protein (APP) or in its processing enzyme result in increased β-site cleavage of APP or favored production of longer, aggregation-prone variants of Aβ peptide [118]. In recent years, however, many studies found that microglia play an important role in the pathogenesis of AD. The reactive gliosis of AD histopathology revealed the abnormal morphology and proliferation of microglia [119, 120]. Several reports have linked microglia dysfunctions to AD, by showing microglial motility impairment in AD mice models [121]. Recently, it was recognized that microglia express voltage-gated ion channels, including Nav1.1, Nav1.5, and Nav1.6 [122, 123]. Furthermore, pharmacological block of the sodium channels has been attempted as a symptomatic treatment of epileptic features often associated with AD, as well as a relief to detrimental behavioral and psychological symptoms of dementia [124]. An interesting debate is if sodium channel activators could just be enough to compensate microglial dysfunctions to altered physiological properties of dysfunctional neuronal networks in AD patients [125].

4.2 Neuroglial sodium channels in Parkinson's disease

PD is the second most common age-related disabling neurodegenerative disorder, estimated to affect over 10 million people worldwide, which PD presents clinically as bradykinesia, muscular rigidity, arresting tremor, and postural stability [126–128]. In addition, PD is characterized by dopamine depletion and the loss of dopaminergic (DA) neurons with accompanying neuroinflammation. The potential causes of PD remain uncertain, but recent studies suggest neuroinflammation and microglia activation play important roles in PD pathogenesis [129, 130]. However, persistent activation of microglia can mediate neuronal death and neurodegeneration by increasing the secretion of inflammatory molecules and cytokines, including tumor necrosis factor alpha (TNF-α) and reactive oxygen species (ROS) [131, 132]. Microglia express a number of ion channels, including sodium channels that regulate various aspects of inflammatory process, providing a potential target for intervention [14, 133]. Several studies demonstrated that VGSC can regulate a number of cellular functions such as morphological transformation, migration, and phagocytosis of microglia [12, 35]. This also indicates the well potential immunomodulatory properties of VGSC. 6-Hydroxydopamine (6-OHDA)-induced PD rat model found that the expressions of Nav1.1, Nav1.3, and Nav1.6 in the hippocampus were dynamically increased at different time points after dopamine depletion. Furthermore, cognitive deficits were effectively improved by phenytoin (sodium channel blocker) that has inhibitory effects on VGSCs in the brain [33]. Other study suggested that zonisamide, targeting VGSCs, may reduce neuroinflammation through the downregulation of microglial Nav 1.6 [134]. Those studies may contribute to its reported neuroprotective role in preclinical models of PD.

5. Application of neuroimaging in studying neuroglial sodium channels

Electrophysiological patch clamp is a classic technique for traditionally recording neuronal sodium channels. Neuroglial cells are non-excitable cells, of which the cell membrane depolarization is not obvious. The bioproperties of neuroglial sodium channels evoked by high voltage in patch clamp recordings might be different from the actual situation in vivo. Therefore, this method has certain limitations in the process of studying neuroglial cells. With the development of ion probes, especially the recent discovery of visible light sodium ion probes as well as calcium ion probes, which could provide more intuitive results (such as higher resolution, better observation) for the functional study of glial cell Nav channels and Nav-NCX complexes [14]. The combined use of ion probes and patch clamping will make the experimental results both more abundant and accurate.

In addition, the invention of the miniature two-photon microscope in 2017 [135] provided a powerful means for the functional research of nerve cells as well as glial cells. During studying brain activities and the development of neuroinflammatory diseases, glial cells could be labeled by GCaMP6 or dTomato to explore the function of the glial Nav-NCX complex. Two-photon imaging combined with EEG could not only explain the relationship between glial cell activity and EEG frequency more effectively, but also elucidate the important role of glial cells in neurological disorders, such as epilepsy. By using the miniature two-photon microscope, the conditional knockout mice could be applied to study the role of glial sodium channels in regulating the function of glial cells or the interaction between glial cells and neurons, including pruning of neuron synapses by microglial cells or regulating the neuroexcitability in vivo.

6. Conclusion

In view of the central role of glia in CNS health and disease, it is necessary to further understand the physiological correlation of glial sodium channels and characterize the molecular pathways that control the function of sodium channels in these cells. There has been much work performed in cell culture, but further in vivo studies are of crucial importance for determination of the therapeutic implications of targeting glial sodium channels in neurological disorders. Therefore, novel neuroimaging techniques are of importance for studying the roles of neuroglial sodium channels in neuroinflammatory diseases. Meanwhile, with the heightened focus on developing sodium channel specific blockers, it is increasingly relevant to assess the roles of individual sodium channel isoforms in neuroglia cells (e.g., Nav1.6 in microglial cells, Nav1.5 in astrocytes). Further understanding of the signaling cascade linking sodium channel activity to glial effector function will facilitate the development of specific therapeutic targets for neurological diseases.

Acknowledgements

This chapter was supported by National Natural Science Foundation of China (Nos. 81603410 and 81903995), Youth Talent Promotion Project of China Association of Chinese Medicine (No. CACM-2019-QNRC2-C10), Shanghai Municipal Commission of Health and Family Planning Fund (Nos. 20184Y0086 and 2018JQ003), Project for Capacity Promotion of Putuo District Clinical Special Disease (2019tszb02), Science and Technology Innovation Project of Putuo District Health System (Nos. ptkwws201902 and ptkwws201908), Project within the Budget of Shanghai University of Traditional Chinese Medicine (Nos. 18-DX-06 and 2019LK040), the Key Speciality Program (No. 2016102A), and Research Project (Nos. 2016208A, 2018302, 2018314, and 2018313) of Putuo Hospital, Shanghai University of Traditional Chinese Medicine.

Conflict of interest

The authors confirm that this article content has no conflict of interest.

Author details

Yu Yao[1,2†], Xiaoli Wang[2†], Shuzhang Zhang[2], Zhiping Zhang[2], Wei Wang[1], Yudan Zhu[1], Jiwei Cheng[1], Guoyi Li[1*] and Jie Tao[1*]

1 Department of Neurology and Central Laboratory, Putuo Hospital, Shanghai University of Traditional Chinese Medicine, Shanghai, China

2 Institute of Biomembrane and Biopharmaceutics, Shanghai University, Shanghai, China

*Address all correspondence to: iliguoyi@163.com and jietao_putuo@foxmail.com

† These authors have contributed equally to this chapter.

References

[1] Huh Y, Ji RR, Chen G. Neuroinflammation, bone marrow stem cells, and chronic pain. Frontiers in Immunology. 2017;**8**:1014. DOI: 10.3389/fimmu.2017.01014

[2] Mayer CL, Huber BR, Peskind E. Traumatic brain injury, neuroinflammation, and post-traumatic headaches. Headache. 2013;**53**(9):1523-1530. DOI: 10.1111/head.12173

[3] Healy LM, Yaqubi M, Ludwin S, et al. Species differences in immune-mediated CNS tissue injury and repair: A (neuro) inflammatory topic. Glia. 2020;**68**(4):811-829

[4] Yang QQ, Zhou JW. Neuroinflammation in the central nervous system: Symphony of glial cells. Glia. 2019;**67**(6):1017-1035. DOI: 10.1002/glia.23571

[5] Wynn TA, Barron L, Thompson RW, et al. Quantitative assessment of macrophage functions in repair and fibrosis. Current Protocols in Immunology. 2011; Chapter 14:Unit14.22. DOI: 10.1002/0471142735.im1422s93

[6] Xiong XY, Liu L, Yang QW. Functions and mechanisms of microglia/macrophages in neuroinflammation and neurogenesis after stroke. Progress in Neurobiology. 2016;**142**:23-44. DOI: 10.1016/j.pneurobio.2016.05.001

[7] Chhor V, Le Charpentier T, Lebon S, et al. Characterization of phenotype markers and neuronotoxic potential of polarised primary microglia in vitro. Brain, Behavior, and Immunity. 2013;**32**:70-85. DOI: 10.1016/j.bbi.2013.02.005

[8] Black JA, Newcombe J, Waxman SG. Astrocytes within multiple sclerosis lesions upregulate sodium channel Nav1.5. Brain: A Journal of Neurology. 2010;**133**(Pt 3):835-846. DOI: 10.1093/brain/awq003

[9] Barateiro A, Brites D, Fernandes A. Oligodendrocyte development and myelination in neurodevelopment: Molecular mechanisms in health and disease. Current Pharmaceutical Design. 2016;**22**(6):656-679. DOI: 10.2174/1381612822666151204000636

[10] Hodgkin AL, Huxley AF. A quantitative description of membrane current and its application to conduction and excitation in nerve. Journal of Physiology. 1952;**117**(4):500-544

[11] Peter M Jr, Hajdu P, Varga Z, et al. Blockage of human T lymphocyte Kv1.3 channels by Pi1, a novel class of scorpion toxin. Biochemical and Biophysical Research Communications. 2000;**278**(1):34-37. DOI: 10.1006/bbrc.2000.3756

[12] Black JA, Liu S, Waxman SG. Sodium channel activity modulates multiple functions in microglia. Glia. 2009;**57**(10):1072-1081. DOI: 10.1002/glia.20830

[13] Craner MJ, Damarjian TG, Liu S, et al. Sodium channels contribute to microglia/macrophage activation and function in EAE and MS. Glia. 2005;**49**(2):220-229. DOI: 10.1002/glia.20112

[14] Pappalardo LW, Black JA, Waxman SG. Sodium channels in astroglia and microglia. Glia. 2016;**64**(10):1628-1645. DOI: 10.1002/glia.22967

[15] Patino GA, Isom LL. Electrophysiology and beyond: Multiple roles of Na^+ channel beta subunits in development and disease. Neuroscience Letters. 2010;**486**(2):53-59. DOI: 10.1016/j.neulet.2010.06.050

[16] Catterall WA. Voltage-gated sodium channels at 60: Structure, function and pathophysiology. The Journal of Physiology. 2012;**590**(11):2577-2589. DOI: 10.1113/jphysiol.2011.224204

[17] Dib-Hajj SD, Cummins TR, Black JA, et al. From genes to pain: Na v 1.7 and human pain disorders. Trends in Neurosciences. 2007;**30**(11):555-563. DOI: 10.1016/j.tins.2007.08.004

[18] Dib-Hajj SD, Yang Y, Black JA, et al. The Na(V)1.7 sodium channel: From molecule to man. Nature Reviews Neuroscience. 2013;**14**(1):49-62. DOI: 10.1038/nrn3404

[19] Wood JN. Ion channels in analgesia research. Handbook of Experimental Pharmacology. 2007;**177**:329-358. DOI: 10.1007/978-3-540-33823-9_12

[20] Hoeijmakers JG, Faber CG, Merkies IS, et al. Painful peripheral neuropathy and sodium channel mutations. Neuroscience Letters. 2015;**596**:51-59. DOI: 10.1016/j.neulet.2014.12.056

[21] Oliva M, Berkovic SF, Petrou S. Sodium channels and the neurobiology of epilepsy (vol 53, pg 1849, 2012). Epilepsia. 2013;**54**(3):570

[22] Waxman SG. Axonal conduction and injury in multiple sclerosis: The role of sodium channels. Nature Reviews Neuroscience. 2006;**7**(12):932-941. DOI: 10.1038/nrn2023

[23] Waxman SG. Mechanisms of disease: Sodium channels and neuroprotection in multiple sclerosis-current status. Nature Clinical Practice Neurology. 2008;**4**(3):159-169. DOI: 10.1038/ncpneuro0735

[24] Nakajima K, Kohsaka S. Microglia: Activation and their significance in the central nervous system. Journal of Biochemistry. 2001;**130**(2):169-175

[25] Ifuku M, Farber K, Okuno Y, et al. Bradykinin-induced microglial migration mediated by B1-bradykinin receptors depends on Ca^{2+} influx via reverse-mode activity of the Na^{+}/Ca^{2+} exchanger. The Journal of Neuroscience: The Official Journal of the Society for Neuroscience. 2007;**27**(48):13065-13073. DOI: 10.1523/jneurosci.3467-07.2007

[26] Noda M, Ifuku M, Mori Y, et al. Calcium influx through reversed NCX controls migration of microglia. Advances in Experimental Medicine and Biology. 2013;**961**:289-294. DOI: 10.1007/978-1-4614-4756-6_24

[27] Ikeda M, Tsuno S, Sugiyama T, et al. Ca(2+) spiking activity caused by the activation of store-operated Ca(2+) channels mediates TNF-alpha release from microglial cells under chronic purinergic stimulation. Biochimica et Biophysica Acta. 2013;**1833**(12):2573-2585. DOI: 10.1016/j.bbamcr.2013.06.022

[28] Annunziato L, Pignataro G, Di Renzo GF. Pharmacology of brain Na^{+}/Ca^{2+} exchanger: From molecular biology to therapeutic perspectives. Pharmacological Reviews. 2004;**56**(4):633-654. DOI: 10.1124/pr.56.4.5

[29] Chatelier A, Zhao J, Bois P, et al. Biophysical characterisation of the persistent sodium current of the Nav1.6 neuronal sodium channel: A single-channel analysis. Pflugers Arch. 2010;**460**(1):77-86

[30] Cheng Y, Zhao J, Qiao W, et al. Recent advances in diagnosis and treatment of gliomas using chlorotoxin-based bioconjugates. American Journal of Nuclear Medicine and Molecular Imaging. 2014;**4**(5):385-405

[31] Pappalardo LW, Samad OA, Liu S, et al. Nav1.5 in astrocytes plays a sex-specific role in clinical outcomes in a mouse model of multiple sclerosis. Glia.

2018;**66**(10):2174-2187. DOI: 10.1002/glia.23470

[32] Black JA, Newcombe J, Trapp BD, et al. Sodium channel expression within chronic multiple sclerosis plaques. Journal of Neuropathology and Experimental Neurology. 2007;**66**(9):828-837. DOI: 10.1097/nen.0b013e3181462841

[33] Wang Z, Lin Y, Liu W, et al. Voltage-gated sodium channels are involved in cognitive impairments in Parkinson's disease-like rats. Neuroscience. 2019;**418**:231-243. DOI: 10.1016/j.neuroscience.2019.08.024

[34] Hossain MM, Blair W, Kenneth R, et al. The anti-parkinsonian drug zonisamide reduces neuroinflammation: Role of microglial Na(v) 1.6. Experimental Neurology. 2018;**308**:111-119

[35] Stevens M, Timmermans S, Bottelbergs A, et al. Block of a subset of sodium channels exacerbates experimental autoimmune encephalomyelitis. Journal of Neuroimmunology. 2013;**261**(1-2):21-28. DOI: 10.1016/j.jneuroim.2013.04.012

[36] Sontheimer H, Black JA, Ransom BR, et al. Ion channels in spinal cord astrocytes in vitro. I. Transient expression of high levels of Na^+ and K^+ channels. Journal of Neurophysiology. 1992;**68**(4):985-1000. DOI: 10.1152/jn.1992.68.4.985

[37] Barres BA, Chun LL, Corey DP. Ion channel expression by white matter glia: I. Type 2 astrocytes and oligodendrocytes. Glia. 1988;**1**(1):10-30. DOI: 10.1002/glia.440010104

[38] Sontheimer H, Perouansky M, Hoppe D, et al. Glial cells of the oligodendrocyte lineage express proton-activated Na+ channels. Journal of Neuroscience Research. 1989;**24**(4):496-500. DOI: 10.1002/jnr.490240406

[39] Kressin K, Kuprijanova E, Jabs R, et al. Developmental regulation of Na^+ and K^+ conductances in glial cells of mouse hippocampal brain slices. Glia. 1995;**15**(2):173-187. DOI: 10.1002/glia.440150210

[40] Chen PH, Cai WQ, Wang LY, et al. A morphological and electrophysiological study on the postnatal development of oligodendrocyte precursor cells in the rat brain. Brain Research. 2008;**1243**:27-37. DOI: 10.1016/j.brainres.2008.09.029

[41] Howe JR, Ritchie JM. Sodium currents in Schwann cells from myelinated and non-myelinated nerves of neonatal and adult rabbits. The Journal of Physiology. 1990;**425**:169-210. DOI: 10.1113/jphysiol.1990.sp018098

[42] Korotzer AR, Cotman CW. Voltage-gated currents expressed by rat microglia in culture. Glia. 1992;**6**(2):81-88. DOI: 10.1002/glia.440060202

[43] Norenberg W, Illes P, Gebicke-Haerter PJ. Sodium channel in isolated human brain macrophages (microglia). Glia. 1994;**10**(3):165-172. DOI: 10.1002/glia.440100303

[44] Fraser SP, Salvador V, Manning EA, et al. Contribution of functional voltage-gated Na^+ channel expression to cell behaviors involved in the metastatic cascade in rat prostate cancer: I. lateral motility. Journal of Cellular Physiology. 2003;**195**(3):479-487. DOI: 10.1002/jcp.10312

[45] Fraser SP, Diss JK, Chioni AM, et al. Voltage-gated sodium channel expression and potentiation of human breast cancer metastasis. Clinical Cancer Research: An Official Journal of the American Association for Cancer

Research. 2005;**11**(15):5381-5389. DOI: 10.1158/1078-0432.ccr-05-0327

[46] Gillet L, Roger S, Besson P, et al. Voltage-gated Sodium Channel activity promotes cysteine Cathepsin-dependent invasiveness and colony growth of human cancer cells. The Journal of Biological Chemistry. 2009;**284**(13):8680-8691. DOI: 10.1074/jbc.M806891200

[47] Nimmerjahn A, Kirchhoff F, Helmchen F. Resting microglial cells are highly dynamic surveillants of brain parenchyma in vivo. Science. 2005;**308**(5726):1314-1318. DOI: 10.1126/science.1110647

[48] Persson AK, Estacion M, Ahn H, et al. Contribution of sodium channels to lamellipodial protrusion and Rac1 and ERK1/2 activation in ATP-stimulated microglia. Glia. 2014;**62**(12):2080-2095. DOI: 10.1002/glia.22728

[49] Kreutzberg GW. Microglia: A sensor for pathological events in the CNS. Trends in Neurosciences. 1996;**19**(8):312-318. DOI: 10.1016/0166-2236(96)10049-7

[50] Davalos D, Grutzendler J, Yang G, et al. ATP mediates rapid microglial response to local brain injury in vivo. Nature Neuroscience. 2005;**8**(6):752-758. DOI: 10.1038/nn1472

[51] Cash E, Rott O. Microglial cells qualify as the stimulators of unprimed CD4+ and CD8+ T lymphocytes in the central nervous system. Clinical and Experimental Immunology. 1994;**98**(2):313-318. DOI: 10.1111/j.1365-2249.1994.tb06143.x

[52] Renno T, Krakowski M, Piccirillo C, et al. TNF-alpha expression by resident microglia and infiltrating leukocytes in the central nervous system of mice with experimental allergic encephalomyelitis. Regulation by Th1 cytokines. Journal of Immunology (Baltimore, MD: 1950). 1995;**154**(2):944-953

[53] Barnett MH, Prineas JW. Relapsing and remitting multiple sclerosis: Pathology of the newly forming lesion. Annals of Neurology. 2004;**55**(4):458-468. DOI: 10.1002/ana.20016

[54] Hoffmann A, Kann O, Ohlemeyer C, et al. Elevation of basal intracellular calcium as a central element in the activation of brain macrophages (microglia): Suppression of receptor-evoked calcium signaling and control of release function. The Journal of Neuroscience: The Official Journal of the Society for Neuroscience. 2003;**23**(11):4410-4419

[55] Kohrman DC, Harris JB, Meisler MH. Mutation detection in the med and medJ alleles of the sodium channel Scn8a. Unusual splicing due to a minor class AT-AC intron. The Journal of Biological Chemistry. 1996;**271**(29):17576-17581. DOI: 10.1074/jbc.271.29.17576

[56] Kettenmann H, Hanisch UK, Noda M, et al. Physiology of microglia. Physiological Reviews. 2011;**91**(2):461-553. DOI: 10.1152/physrev.00011.2010

[57] Ridley AJ. Membrane ruffling and signal transduction. BioEssays: News and Reviews in Molecular, Cellular and Developmental Biology. 1994;**16**(5):321-327. DOI: 10.1002/bies.950160506

[58] Honda S, Sasaki Y, Ohsawa K, et al. Extracellular ATP or ADP induce chemotaxis of cultured microglia through Gi/o-coupled P2Y receptors. The Journal of Neuroscience: The Official Journal of the Society for Neuroscience. 2001;**21**(6):1975-1982

[59] Siddiqui TA, Lively S, Vincent C, et al. Regulation of podosome formation, microglial migration and invasion by Ca(2+)-signaling molecules expressed in podosomes. Journal of Neuroinflammation. 2012;**9**:250. DOI: 10.1186/1742-2094-9-250

[60] Ridley AJ, Paterson HF, Johnston CL, et al. The small GTP-binding protein rac regulates growth factor-induced membrane ruffling. Cell. 1992;**70**(3):401-410. DOI: 10.1016/0092-8674(92)90164-8

[61] Huang C, Jacobson K, Schaller MD. MAP kinases and cell migration. Journal of Cell Science. 2004;**117**(Pt 20):4619-4628. DOI: 10.1242/jcs.01481

[62] Wei C, Wang X, Zheng M, et al. Calcium gradients underlying cell migration. Current Opinion in Cell Biology. 2012;**24**(2):254-261. DOI: 10.1016/j.ceb.2011.12.002

[63] Aspenstrom P. Integration of signalling pathways regulated by small GTPases and calcium. Biochimica et Biophysica Acta. 2004;**1742**(1-3):51-58. DOI: 10.1016/j.bbamcr.2004.09.029

[64] Schwab A, Fabian A, Hanley PJ, et al. Role of ion channels and transporters in cell migration. Physiological Reviews. 2012;**92**(4):1865-1913. DOI: 10.1152/physrev.00018.2011

[65] Chuderland D, Marmor G, Shainskaya A, et al. Calcium-mediated interactions regulate the subcellular localization of extracellular signal-regulated kinases. The Journal of Biological Chemistry. 2008;**283**(17):11176-11188. DOI: 10.1074/jbc.M709030200

[66] Bisi S, Disanza A, Malinverno C, et al. Membrane and actin dynamics interplay at lamellipodia leading edge. Current Opinion in Cell Biology. 2013;**25**(5):565-573. DOI: 10.1016/j.ceb.2013.04.001

[67] Ridley AJ. Life at the leading edge. Cell. 2011;**145**(7):1012-1022. DOI: 10.1016/j.cell.2011.06.010

[68] Dong Y, Benveniste EN. Immune function of astrocytes. Glia. 2001;**36**(2):180-190. DOI: 10.1002/glia.1107

[69] Prat A, Antel J. Pathogenesis of multiple sclerosis. Current Opinion in Neurology. 2005;**18**(3):225-230. DOI: 10.1097/01.wco.0000169737.99040.31

[70] Nair A, Frederick TJ, Miller SD. Astrocytes in multiple sclerosis: A product of their environment. Cellular and Molecular Life Sciences. 2008;**65**(17):2702-2720. DOI: 10.1007/s00018-008-8059-5

[71] Pappalardo LW, Liu S, Black JA, et al. Dynamics of sodium channel Nav1.5 expression in astrocytes in mouse models of multiple sclerosis. Neuroreport. 2014;**25**(15):1208-1215. DOI: 10.1097/wnr.0000000000000249

[72] Sontheimer H, Black JA, Waxman SG. Voltage-gated Na^+ channels in glia: Properties and possible functions. Trends in Neurosciences. 1996;**19**(8):325-331. DOI: 10.1016/0166-2236(96)10039-4

[73] Black JA, Dib-Hajj S, Cohen S, et al. Glial cells have heart: rH1 Na^+ channel mRNA and protein in spinal cord astrocytes. Glia. 1998;**23**(3):200-208

[74] Pappalardo LW, Samad OA, Black JA, et al. Voltage-gated sodium channel Nav 1.5 contributes to astrogliosis in an in vitro model of glial injury via reverse Na^+/Ca^{2+} exchange. Glia. 2014;**62**(7):1162-1175. DOI: 10.1002/glia.22671

[75] Macfarlane SN, Sontheimer H. Spinal cord astrocytes display a switch from TTX-sensitive to TTX-resistant sodium currents after injury-induced gliosis in vitro. Journal of Neurophysiology. 1998;**79**(4):2222-2226. DOI: 10.1152/jn.1998.79.4.2222

[76] Thio CL, Sontheimer H. Differential modulation of TTX-sensitive and TTX-resistant Na+ channels in spinal cord astrocytes following activation of protein kinase C. The Journal of Neuroscience: The Official Journal

of the Society for Neuroscience. 1993;**13**(11):4889-4897

[77] Kastritsis CH, Salm AK, McCarthy K. Stimulation of the P2Y purinergic receptor on type 1 astroglia results in inositol phosphate formation and calcium mobilization. Journal of Neurochemistry. 1992;**58**(4):1277-1284. DOI: 10.1111/j.1471-4159.1992.tb11339.x

[78] Parnis J, Montana V, Delgado-Martinez I, et al. Mitochondrial exchanger NCLX plays a major role in the intracellular Ca^{2+} signaling, gliotransmission, and proliferation of astrocytes. The Journal of Neuroscience: The Official Journal of the Society for Neuroscience. 2013;**33**(17):7206-7219. DOI: 10.1523/jneurosci.5721-12.2013

[79] Gao K, Wang CR, Jiang F, et al. Traumatic scratch injury in astrocytes triggers calcium influx to activate the JNK/c-Jun/AP-1 pathway and switch on GFAP expression. Glia. 2013;**61**(12):2063-2077. DOI: 10.1002/glia.22577

[80] Stanimirovic DB, Ball R, Mealing G, et al. The role of intracellular calcium and protein kinase C in endothelin-stimulated proliferation of rat type I astrocytes. Glia. 1995;**15**(2):119-130. DOI: 10.1002/glia.440150204

[81] Wang HH, Hsieh HL, Yang CM. Calmodulin kinase II-dependent transactivation of PDGF receptors mediates astrocytic MMP-9 expression and cell motility induced by lipoteichoic acid. Journal of Neuroinflammation. 2010;7:84. DOI: 10.1186/1742-2094-7-84

[82] Reyes RC, Verkhratsky A, Parpura V. Plasmalemmal Na^{+}/Ca^{2+} exchanger modulates Ca^{2+}-dependent exocytotic release of glutamate from rat cortical astrocytes. ASN Neuro. 2012;**4**(1):e00075

[83] Kirischuk S, Kettenmann H, Verkhratsky A. Na^{+}/Ca^{2+} exchanger modulates kainate-triggered Ca^{2+} signaling in Bergmann glial cells in situ. FASEB Journal: Official Publication of the Federation of American Societies for Experimental Biology. 1997;**11**(7):566-572. DOI: 10.1096/fasebj.11.7.9212080

[84] Floyd CL, Gorin FA, Lyeth BG. Mechanical strain injury increases intracellular sodium and reverses Na^{+}/Ca^{2+} exchange in cortical astrocytes. Glia. 2005;**51**(1):35-46. DOI: 10.1002/glia.20183

[85] Black JA, Liu S, Carrithers M, et al. Exacerbation of experimental autoimmune encephalomyelitis after withdrawal of phenytoin and carbamazepine. Annals of Neurology. 2007;**62**(1):21-33. DOI: 10.1002/ana.21172

[86] Bechtold DA, Miller SJ, Dawson AC, et al. Axonal protection achieved in a model of multiple sclerosis using lamotrigine. Journal of Neurology. 2006;**253**(12):1542-1551. DOI: 10.1007/s00415-006-0204-1

[87] Morsali D, Bechtold D, Lee W, et al. Safinamide and flecainide protect axons and reduce microglial activation in models of multiple sclerosis. Brain: A Journal of Neurology. 2013;**136**(Pt 4):1067-1082. DOI: 10.1093/brain/awt041

[88] Small RK, Riddle P, Noble M. Evidence for migration of oligodendrocyte--type-2 astrocyte progenitor cells into the developing rat optic nerve. Nature. 1987;**328**(6126):155-157. DOI: 10.1038/328155a0

[89] Menn B, Garcia-Verdugo JM, Yaschine C, et al. Origin of oligodendrocytes in the subventricular zone of the adult brain. The Journal of Neuroscience: The Official Journal of the Society for Neuroscience. 2006;**26**(30):7907-7918. DOI: 10.1523/jneurosci.1299-06.2006

[90] Chang A, Nishiyama A, Peterson J, et al. NG2-positive oligodendrocyte

progenitor cells in adult human brain and multiple sclerosis lesions. The Journal of Neuroscience: The Official Journal of the Society for Neuroscience. 2000;**20**(17):6404-6412

[91] Aguirre A, Dupree JL, Mangin JM, et al. A functional role for EGFR signaling in myelination and remyelination. Nature Neuroscience. 2007;**10**(8):990-1002. DOI: 10.1038/nn1938

[92] Karadottir R, Hamilton NB, Bakiri Y, et al. Spiking and nonspiking classes of oligodendrocyte precursor glia in CNS white matter. Nature Neuroscience. 2008;**11**(4):450-456. DOI: 10.1038/nn2060

[93] Tong XP, Li XY, Zhou B, et al. Ca(2+) signaling evoked by activation of Na(+) channels and Na(+)/Ca(2+) exchangers is required for GABA-induced NG2 cell migration. The Journal of Cell Biology. 2009;**186**(1):113-128. DOI: 10.1083/jcb.200811071

[94] Heng JI, Moonen G, Nguyen L. Neurotransmitters regulate cell migration in the telencephalon. The European Journal of Neuroscience. 2007;**26**(3):537-546. DOI: 10.1111/j.1460-9568.2007.05694.x

[95] Patel DC, Tewari BP, Chaunsali L, et al. Neuron-glia interactions in the pathophysiology of epilepsy. Nature Reviews Neuroscience. 2019;**20**(5):282-297. DOI: 10.1038/s41583-019-0126-4

[96] Meyer AC, Dua T, Ma J, et al. Global disparities in the epilepsy treatment gap: A systematic review. Bulletin of the World Health Organization. 2010;**88**(4):260-266. DOI: 10.2471/blt.09.064147

[97] Liddelow SA, Guttenplan KA, Clarke LE, et al. Neurotoxic reactive astrocytes are induced by activated microglia. Nature. 2017;**541**(7638):481-487. DOI: 10.1038/nature21029

[98] Sofroniew MV. Astrogliosis. Cold Spring Harbor Perspectives in Biology. 2014;**7**(2):a020420. DOI: 10.1101/cshperspect.a020420

[99] Robel S, Buckingham SC, Boni JL, et al. Reactive astrogliosis causes the development of spontaneous seizures. The Journal of Neuroscience: The Official Journal of the Society for Neuroscience. 2015;**35**(8):3330-3345. DOI: 10.1523/jneurosci.1574-14.2015

[100] Olsen ML, Sontheimer H. Functional implications for Kir4.1 channels in glial biology: From K^+ buffering to cell differentiation. Journal of Neurochemistry. 2008;**107**(3):589-601. DOI: 10.1111/j.1471-4159.2008.05615.x

[101] Izquierdo P, Attwell D, Madry C. Ion channels and receptors as determinants of microglial function. Trends in Neurosciences. 2019;**42**(4):278-292. DOI: 10.1016/j.tins.2018.12.007

[102] Sasaki Y, Ohsawa K, Kanazawa H, et al. Iba1 is an actin-cross-linking protein in macrophages/microglia. Biochemical and Biophysical Research Communications. 2001;**286**(2):292-297. DOI: 10.1006/bbrc.2001.5388

[103] Kaplan DI, Isom LL, Petrou S. Role of sodium channels in epilepsy. Cold Spring Harbor Perspectives in Medicine. 2016;**6**(6):a022814

[104] Kwong K, Carr MJ. Voltage-gated sodium channels. Current Opinion in Pharmacology. 2015;**22**:131-139. DOI: 10.1016/j.coph.2015.04.007

[105] Morin-Brureau M, Milior G, Royer J, et al. Microglial phenotypes in the human epileptic temporal lobe. Brain: A Journal of Neurology. 2018;**141**(12):3343-3360. DOI: 10.1093/brain/awy276

[106] Heinemann U, Lux HD. Ceiling of stimulus induced rises in

extracellular potassium concentration in the cerebral cortex of cat. Brain Research. 1977;**120**(2):231-249. DOI: 10.1016/0006-8993(77)90903-9

[107] Steinhauser C, Seifert G. Glial membrane channels and receptors in epilepsy: Impact for generation and spread of seizure activity. European Journal of Pharmacology. 2002;**447**(2-3):227-237. DOI: 10.1016/s0014-2999(02)01846-0

[108] Zhu H, Zhao Y, Wu H, et al. Remarkable alterations of Nav1.6 in reactive astrogliosis during epileptogenesis. Scientific Reports. 2016;**6**:38108. DOI: 10.1038/srep38108

[109] Qiao X, Werkman TR, Gorter JA, et al. Expression of sodium channel alpha subunits 1.1, 1.2 and 1.6 in rat hippocampus after kainic acid-induced epilepsy. Epilepsy Research. 2013;**106**(1-2):17-28. DOI: 10.1016/j.eplepsyres.2013.06.006

[110] Uebachs M, Opitz T, Royeck M, et al. Efficacy loss of the anticonvulsant carbamazepine in mice lacking sodium channel beta subunits via paradoxical effects on persistent sodium currents. The Journal of Neuroscience: The Official Journal of the Society for Neuroscience. 2010;**30**(25):8489-8501. DOI: 10.1523/jneurosci.1534-10.2010

[111] Gorter JA, van Vliet EA, Lopes da Silva FH, et al. Sodium channel beta1-subunit expression is increased in reactive astrocytes in a rat model for mesial temporal lobe epilepsy. European Journal of Neuroscience. 2002;**16**(2):360-364

[112] Aronica E, Yankaya B, Troost D, et al. Induction of neonatal sodium channel II and III alpha-isoform mRNAs in neurons and microglia after status epilepticus in the rat hippocampus. The European Journal of Neuroscience. 2001;**13**(6):1261-1266. DOI: 10.1046/j.0953-816x.2001.01502.x

[113] Gorter JA, Zurolo E, Iyer A, et al. Induction of sodium channel Na(x) (SCN7A) expression in rat and human hippocampus in temporal lobe epilepsy. Epilepsia. 2010;**51**(9):1791-1800. DOI: 10.1111/j.1528-1167.2010.02678.x

[114] James BD, Leurgans SE, Hebert LE, et al. Contribution of Alzheimer disease to mortality in the United States. Neurology. 2014;**82**(12):1045-1050. DOI: 10.1212/WNL.0000000000000240

[115] Weuve J, Hebert LE, Scherr PA, et al. Deaths in the United States among persons with Alzheimer's disease (2010-2050). Alzheimer's & Dementia: The Journal of the Alzheimer's Association. 2014;**10**(2):e40-e46. DOI: 10.1016/j.jalz.2014.01.004

[116] Villemagne VL, Burnham S, Bourgeat P, et al. Amyloid beta deposition, neurodegeneration, and cognitive decline in sporadic Alzheimer's disease: A prospective cohort study. Lancet Neurology. 2013;**12**(4):357-367. DOI: 10.1016/s1474-4422(13)70044-9

[117] Fleisher AS, Chen K, Quiroz YT, et al. Florbetapir PET analysis of amyloid-beta deposition in the presenilin 1 E280A autosomal dominant Alzheimer's disease kindred: A cross-sectional study. Lancet Neurology. 2012;**11**(12):1057-1065. DOI: 10.1016/s1474-4422(12)70227-2

[118] Selkoe DJ, Hardy J. The amyloid hypothesis of Alzheimer's disease at 25 years. EMBO Molecular Medicine. 2016;**8**(6):595-608. DOI: 10.15252/emmm.201606210

[119] Ransohoff RM, Perry VH. Microglial physiology: Unique stimuli, specialized responses. Annual Review of Immunology. 2009;**27**:119-145. DOI: 10.1146/annurev.immunol.021908.132528

[120] Glass CK, Saijo K, Winner B, et al. Mechanisms underlying inflammation

in neurodegeneration. Cell. 2010;**140**(6):918-934. DOI: 10.1016/j.cell.2010.02.016

[121] Krabbe G, Halle A, Matyash V, et al. Functional impairment of microglia coincides with Beta-amyloid deposition in mice with Alzheimer-like pathology. PLoS One. 2013;**8**(4):e60921. DOI: 10.1371/journal.pone.0060921

[122] Kagan BL, Hirakura Y, Azimov R, et al. The channel hypothesis of Alzheimer's disease: Current status. Peptides. 2002;**23**(7):1311-1315. DOI: 10.1016/s0196-9781(02)00067-0

[123] Black JA, Frezel N, Dib-Hajj SD, et al. Expression of Nav1.7 in DRG neurons extends from peripheral terminals in the skin to central preterminal branches and terminals in the dorsal horn. Molecular Pain. 2012;**8**:82. DOI: 10.1186/1744-8069-8-82

[124] Palop JJ, Mucke L. Amyloid-beta-induced neuronal dysfunction in Alzheimer's disease: From synapses toward neural networks. Nature Neuroscience. 2010;**13**(7):812-818. DOI: 10.1038/nn.2583

[125] Jensen HS, Grunnet M, Bastlund JF. Therapeutic potential of Na(V)1.1 activators. Trends in Pharmacological Sciences. 2014;**35**(3):113-118. DOI: 10.1016/j.tips.2013.12.007

[126] Dorsey ER, Constantinescu R, Thompson JP, et al. Projected number of people with Parkinson disease in the most populous nations, 2005 through 2030. Neurology. 2007;**68**(5):384-386. DOI: 10.1212/01.wnl.0000247740.47667.03

[127] Bennett JP. Free radicals, oxidative stress and the origin of Parkinson's disease. Journal of the Neurological Sciences. 1999;**170**(2):75-76. DOI: 10.1016/s0022-510x(99)00191-4

[128] Richardson JR, Hossain MM. Microglial ion channels as potential targets for neuroprotection in Parkinson's disease. Neural Plasticity. 2013;**2013**:587418. DOI: 10.1155/2013/587418

[129] Tansey MG, Goldberg MS. Neuroinflammation in Parkinson's disease: Its role in neuronal death and implications for therapeutic intervention. Neurobiology of Disease. 2010;**37**(3):510-518. DOI: 10.1016/j.nbd.2009.11.004

[130] Wang Q, Liu Y, Zhou J. Neuroinflammation in Parkinson's disease and its potential as therapeutic target. Translational Neurodegeneration. 2015;**4**:19. DOI: 10.1186/s40035-015-0042-0

[131] Harrigan TJ, Abdullaev IF, Jourd'heuil D, et al. Activation of microglia with zymosan promotes excitatory amino acid release via volume-regulated anion channels: The role of NADPH oxidases. Journal of Neurochemistry. 2008;**106**(6):2449-2462. DOI: 10.1111/j.1471-4159.2008.05553.x

[132] Liu Y, Kintner DB, Chanana V, et al. Activation of microglia depends on Na^+/H^+ exchange-mediated H^+ homeostasis. The Journal of Neuroscience: The Official Journal of the Society for Neuroscience. 2010;**30**(45):15210-15220. DOI: 10.1523/jneurosci.3950-10.2010

[133] Hossain MM, Liu J, Richardson JR. Pyrethroid insecticides directly activate microglia through interaction with voltage-gated sodium channels. Toxicological Sciences: An Official Journal of the Society of Toxicology. 2017;**155**(1):112-123. DOI: 10.1093/toxsci/kfw187

[134] Hossain MM, Weig B, Reuhl K, et al. The anti-parkinsonian drug zonisamide reduces neuroinflammation:

Role of microglial Nav 1.6. Experimental Neurology. 2018;**308**:111-119. DOI: 10.1016/j.expneurol.2018.07.005

[135] Zong W, Wu R, Li M, et al. Fast high-resolution miniature two-photon microscopy for brain imaging in freely behaving mice. Nature Methods. 2017;**14**(7):713-719. DOI: 10.1038/nmeth.4305

Chapter 2

Hypothalamic-Pituitary-Adrenal (HPA) Axis and Chronic Fatigue Syndrome in Older Adults: The Rehabilitation Perspectives

Frank Ho-Yin Lai, Maria Uscinska and Elaine Wai-hung Yan

Abstract

Chronic fatigue syndrome (CFS) is a long-term and debilitating condition that regards as a neurological disease. Its symptoms include profound physical and mental fatigue (characteristically made worse by exertion), muscle and joint pain, disturbed sleep, and both concentration and memory problems. CFS is a kind of human stress-related disorders that are characterized by alterations in hypothalamic-pituitary-adrenal (HPA) axis activity. Investigation of abnormal activity of the HPA axis in various neurological and neuropsychiatric disorders can date back at least 60 years, and its relation to CFS had been reported in the early 1990s. This chapter further disseminated updated evidence for disruption of HPA function in CFS, with the explanation on the relationship between cytokines and HPA activities. Moreover, very limited literature had addressed the importance of rehabilitation to them . This chapter addresses this gap by sharing a pilot rehabilitation outcome on a single-blinded randomized control trial with a parallel group experimental design in the application of activity scheduling (AS) program of occupational therapy for a group of community-dwelling older adults with CFS. The primary objective is to study the outcome of physical functioning of individual participants. The second objective is to study the outcome of AS on impact of caring role through assessing individual caregivers' perceived burden in care. The third objective is to study the time that needed in taking care; individuals' perception of enjoyment and achievement in their participated activities will be evaluated. There was a significant effect of AS on the physical functioning of participants as measured by Functional Independence Measure (FIM), as the primary outcome measure, in experimental group, with Wilk's $\lambda = 0.72$, $F\ (2,57) = 18.75$, $p < 0.001$. Moreover, in secondary outcome measures, there is a significant decrease in the impact of caring role as reflected by their perceived burden as measured by the Chinese Zarit Burden Interview (CZBI) in caring for experimental group, with Wilk's $\lambda = 0.72$, $F\ (2,97) = 18.75$, $p < 0.001$. Another study set out to examine the effect of time on caring activities for those recruited couples in AS group. There was significant effect of AS on caring activities with Wilk's $\lambda = 0.71$, $F\ (2,97) = 12.47$, $p < 0.001$. With proper coaching and regular facilitation regarding AS, activity participation in older adults with CFS can be greatly enhanced. Behavioral intervention, such as AS, can supplement therapeutic treatment or may lead to decline in CFS symptoms.

IntechOpen

Keywords: chronic fatigue syndrome (CFS), hypothalamic-pituitary-adrenal (HPA) axis, activity scheduling (AS)

1. Introduction

There are two perspectives in developing this chapter [1–3]. The first perspective is to provide an up-to-date and intensive literature search in analyzing the physiological, neurological, and molecular factors that lead to chronic fatigue syndrome (CFS). This part will provide the reader with background information on the importance of neuroimaging, clinical relationship between CFS and hypothalamic-pituitary-adrenal (HPA) axis, and its physiological causes with different cytokines. The second perspective addresses the impact of CFS to individuals' life role through the behavioral intervention by activity scheduling (AS). Its effectiveness was examined by a single-blinded randomized control trial with a parallel group experimental design.

CFS is a complex illness characterized by a broad range of physiological, cognitive, neurological, and emotional symptoms [4]. The signs and symptoms of CFS include fatigue, loss of concentration, unexplained muscle or joint pain, headache, unrefreshing sleep, and extreme exhaustion [5]. It continues to evolve as a disabling phenomenon characterized by debilitating fatigue and consequential components that limit the functional ability of persons afflicted with the disease [6]. One important theory in the cause of CFS is the deficits in the central nervous system and HPA in short [4, 7, 8].

1.1 Biomedical marker: neuroimaging

The proper diagnosis of CFS should come with specific biomedical markers, such as neuroimaging, in order to confirm with the subjective information, signs, and symptoms provided by the patient in order to make the proper clinical diagnosis with strong clinical definition of this syndrome [9]. Reported cognitive difficulties and complaints of headache can be scientifically reviewed by brain imaging [10]. Three neuroimaging approaches have been commonly used clinically. The first of these is the functional magnetic resonance imaging (fMRI), which allows researchers to look at where in the brain activation is associated with a task or an experience [11, 12]. The diffusion tensor imaging (DTI) enables researchers to look at the health of the brain's white matter [13], and *voxel-based morphometry* (VBM) allows researchers to investigate structural changes in the brain [14, 15]. These three approaches were used to scientifically examine by imaging on how likely it was for the reported fatigue from patients. Moreover, a number of well-cited correlational studies between neuroimaging and clinical measurements showed the strong evidence in applying neuroimaging [16] and particularly for CFS [17]. There was a significant negative correlation between micro-structural integration, such as radial kurtosis, reflecting biological microenvironment imaging metric in the hypothalamus [17, 18] and fatigue-related scale in traumatic patients [19].

1.2 Relationship between CFS and HPA

Symptoms of CFS include persistent fatigue, difficulty with memory and concentration, a disturbed sleep pattern, and severe musculoskeletal pain [20]. The symptoms displayed vary from individuals; some may need to remain bed rest for long periods of time [8], while others are able to manage their fatigue by maintaining their own activities of daily living [3]. CFS presents with symptoms and abnormalities of HPA [21]. The HPA axis dysregulation may have a causal role in CFS [1, 19, 22]. Diagnosis is difficult because there is no diagnostic marker for the disease and no standard test; rather, a diagnosis is based on the description and duration of symptoms [2], degree of impairment [7], and clinical findings that rule out other diseases [23]. The effect on lifestyle and self-image are considerable because of significant changes in participation in activities, identity, and occupational issues [24].

Dysregulation of the biological systems which mediate the response to stress potentially has an important role in the etiopathogenesis of CFS [25, 26]. The neurobiological stress system comprises a range of networks that form intricate pathways; an important part of this is the HPA axis [27, 28] which is a self-regulated feedback system which contributes to the maintenance of homeostasis and which is impacted by multiple factors such as time of day and physical and psychological stressors [20]. CFS is a debilitating illness which was classified as a neurological disease [29]. Experimentally induced, or pathological, hypocortisolemia (as in Addison's disease) is associated with symptoms typical of CFS, including fatigue, weakness, and abdominal pain, but it is also associated with a range of other features which are not typical of CFS [30]. Inactivity, sleep disturbance, psychiatric comorbidity, medication, and ongoing stress experienced by people with CFS will affect HPA axis function [1, 28, 31, 32], and the findings that HPA axis dysregulation is more prominent in patients with a longer duration of illness suggest that the endocrine changes may be secondary [33, 34]. Researchers further supported that the individual variation in HPA axis regulation in patients with CFS argues for a heterogeneous and multifactorial bidirectional relationship between the endocrine disturbance and the disorder [35].

1.3 Physiological causes of CFS

Feelings of fatigue are common symptoms associated with infectious diseases and many other physical [36] and mental pathologic conditions [37]. Since the early 1990s, there has been a systematic study on changes in CFS that occur with infection or following microbial product-induced cytokine production in relation to CFS [38–40]. Moreover, research has shown a strong interaction between the HPA axis and the immune system [41, 42]. Some cytokines have stimulating effect on the HPA axis, whereas cortisol, the end product of the HPA axis, suppresses secretion. Elevated tumor necrosis factor α (TNFα), interleukin-2 (IL-2), and/or interleukin-6 (IL-6) levels may be the mediators of fatigue associated with primary or secondary adrenal insufficiency.

1.4 Tumor necrosis factor α

TNFα is an inflammatory cytokine that is predominantly produced by activated macrophages. In addition, TNFα is also expressed by other immune cells (lymphoid cells, mast cells, fibroblasts) as well as endothelial cells and nerve cells. TNFα is a key signaling molecule for cell death process (by activation of NF-κB and JNK-MAPK pathways). Therefore, TNFα may indicate pathological mechanisms of numerous diseases, including neural degeneration common to neurocognitive disorders. Indeed, TNFα has been associated with Alzheimer's disease and mild cognitive impairments. Increased levels of TNFα have been found in serum and CSF [43], as well as postmortem brain tissues [44] of Alzheimer's disease patients compared with control subjects. Moreover, the elevation in TNF was apparent before the emergence of overt cognitive deficits [44]. Its potential as an early marker therefore certainly warrants investigation, especially from a longitudinal perspective. TNFα secretion in young adults showed a statistically significant circadian rhythm with a peak close to the offset of sleep [45]; such a rhythm was not present in older adults [46].

1.5 Interleukin-6

IL-6 is a pleiotropic cytokine released by a host of immune cells (T cells and monocytes) [47], and it plays a critical role in the regulation of the inflammatory responses in the host immune defense. Specifically, IL-6 stimulates B-cell differentiation and antibody production. Higher levels of IL-6 are associated with various autoimmune and inflammatory diseases. The risk of a decline in Mini-Mental State Examination (MMSE) over a 10-year period is higher among people with higher IL-6 levels (odds ratio = 1.81, $CI_{95\%}$, 1.20, 2.71) [48]. The same study also showed that IL-6 levels predicted the magnitude of 10-year decline in reasoning (high IL-6, 20.35; $CI_{95\%}$, 20.37, 20.33 vs. low IL-6, 20.29; $CI_{95\%}$, 20.31, 20.27). Through synergistic interaction with other cytokines, IL-6 also regulates platelet production by bone marrow cells (via synergy with IL-3-regulated megakaryocyte development), secretion of acute-phase proteins by liver cells (via synergy with IL-1), and bone homeostasis (e.g., via RANKL-mediated mechanism) [48].

IL-6 in humans caused profound somnolence and fatigue [49]. Literature reviewed the decrease in overall secretion of IL-6 is associated with a good sleep that is associated with decreased exposure of tissues to the proinflammatory [50] and potentially detrimental actions of IL-6 on the cardiovascular system, insulin sensitivity, and bones [51–53].

1.6 Adrenal insufficiency

Adrenal insufficiency is associated also with chronic fatigue [4, 54]. Previous studies indicated that untreated patients with adrenal insufficiency demonstrated increased sleep fragmentation [55, 56], findings that may explain the patients' fatigue. These sleep abnormalities were reversed following treatment with a replacement dose of hydrocortisone. These results suggest that cortisol secretion may be needed to facilitate both initiation and maintenance of REM sleep. It should be noted that in normal individuals, exogenous glucocorticoids have been found to reduce REM sleep [57]. Behaviorally, excessive daytime sleepiness is prominent in patients with secondary adrenal insufficiency [58].

1.7 Impact of CFS to individuals' life roles

Fatigue, a poorly defined phenomenon and subjective in nature, was described by CFS sufferers as continuous, resulting in diminished engagement in activities [59]. It was found that most individuals with CFS actually underreported their disabilities [6]. Moreover, functional limitations consequently affect the successful completion of tasks and roles [3]. The loss or diminishment of these roles as providers, family members, and peers affects not only functional relationships but also the quality of life of their partners, family members, and significant others [60, 61].

1.8 Intervention

Because the etiology of CFS is unidentified, the relief of symptoms is the primary goal when treating this population. Previously, the effectiveness of many of the treatments was unproven (Berne, 2002). Nowadays, apart from pharmacological interventions [62, 63], some directions were shown to be effective, like nutrition [64] and use of exercise [65–68] and cognitive behavioral therapy [69, 70]. The general consensus was that graded exercise therapy (GET), cognitive behavioral therapy (CBT), and "pacing" (energy conservation) showed the most positive results.

1.9 Consideration of rehabilitation for CFS

Literature has shown behavioral intervention can supplement therapeutic treatment [71] or may lead to decline in CFS symptoms [72, 73]. Occupational therapy addresses problems for those individuals at risk or already experiencing problems in performing activities that affect functional independence, health, and wellbeing due to accident, illness, or delays [3]. As a holistic practice, occupational therapy addresses individuals' physical, social, and psychological areas of life. Much has been contributed by occupational therapists to populations with chronic disease and populations with fatigue, loss of concentration, unexplained musculoskeletal pain, and amotivational symptoms that are similar to CFS [6]. The focus of occupational therapy is placed on individuals' meaningful participation of activities [74]. This may act as structuring the engagement in activities of older adults need to do (self-care), enjoy doing (leisure), and do for progress (productivity) and help them to develop a sense of self-worth and wellbeing [75–78].

Activity scheduling is a tailor-made personalized activity that can be used as a media for behavioral activation [79, 80]. AS is the technique that compromise the advantages of GET, CBT, and energy conservation techniques. It has been established as a core component of evidence-based treatment for depression with equivalent outcomes to cognitive behavioral therapy [81], through introducing small and easily achievable changes, gradually building up levels of activity toward individualized short-term to long-term goals [80]. In their meta-analysis on randomized effect studies of AS, 16 studies with 780 subjects were included. The pooled effect size indicating the difference between AS intervention and control conditions yield a large effect size of 0.87 (95% CI, 0.60–1.15). Moreover, there was a robust association between AS during treatment and self-reported activity engagement as well as clinically significant improvements in depression [82, 83]. AS is an effective behavioral intervention that can address social isolation in older adults [83, 84]. Older adults can experience higher degrees of engagement in social activities, more chances to experience positive emotions [83], and a sense of not being negatively affected or neglected in their limited interactions with their environments [85]. Moreover, AS has been shown to be effective in enhancing individuals' quality of life through increasing their active participation in activities [80, 82].

This study is a pioneer attempt to examine if AS would show its effectiveness in the management of older adults whom suffered from CFS. The primary objective is to study the outcome of physical functioning of individual participants. The second objective is to study the outcome on impact of caring role through assessing individual caregivers' perceived burden in care. The third objective is to study the time that needed in taking care and individuals' perception of enjoyment and achievement in their participated activities.

2. Methods

This 10-week longitudinal study was a single-blinded randomized control trial with a parallel group experimental design.

2.1 Participants

Older adults with CFS and their spouse caregivers would be recruited. Both of them should be age-ranged from 65 to 70 years. Participants with CFS should have a diagnosis in their medical history under the ICD-10 criteria which was diagnosed by a physician. Individuals' cognitive function would be screened by the Montreal Cognitive Assessment Hong Kong Version (MoCA-HK) [86]. To ensure participants having intact cognitive function, both participants with CFS and their spouse caregivers would be screened with MoCA-HK and should have a score >26. After provision of clear verbal and written explanation on the purpose of this study, they will provide their consent with the presence of their social workers. Approval was given by the local research ethics committee, and the study was conducted according to the Declaration of Helsinki.

2.2 Interventions

Participants with CFS and their spouse caregivers in both groups received a health education program with weekly themed topics, such as the importance of exercise and healthy eating, sleep management, counseling, acceptance therapy, and commitment therapy in the first and second weeks. For the following 8 weeks, they would be randomized and received one of the two interventions. Healthcare Education group, as control group, would receive eight weekly education sessions on health and physical care education offered by lecturers of occupational therapy from a local university. In experimental arm, Healthcare Education-Activity Scheduling (Healthcare ED-AS group) would receive the same health and physical care education program and AS training, focusing on pleasant activities and improving communication.

After receiving three-session training from two occupational therapists, AS became a caregiver-delivered intervention, and it involves five steps: (1) baseline assessment, (2) discussion, (3) homework, (4) enhancing motivation and encouragement, and (5) reassessment. Moreover, those two occupational therapists who conducted the training would provide weekly telephone follow-up for caregivers as the strategy in encouraging individuals' completion of program.

In the baseline assessment, researcher interviewed each couple in their own home. The occupational therapist would document the activities pattern of older adults over the course of a week. For each activity, participants should rate their own sense of enjoyment (E) and achievement (A) between 0 and 10 ("0" = no sense of enjoyment or achievement and "10" = you enjoyed the activity very much or felt a strong sense of achievement). Participants would mark this immediately after completing the activity or at the end of the day. Moreover, measures on the amount of time in taking care and individuals' perception of enjoyment and achievement in their participated activities would serve as the baseline reading of their current activity levels. In discussion, activities chosen in AS had to be related on what the participants had been avoiding and help them to act in accordance with their valued directions. Spouse caregivers were asked to monitor the mood when they participated in their scheduled activities. They would be evaluated whether or not what they did was in keeping with their goals and valued directions. They were encouraged to make notes, and the occupational therapist would provide regular support in regard to assessing areas that were still avoided and activities that are overused. In homework, spouse caregivers could use the activity achievement worksheet to indicate how they spent their time, as well as how the activities affected their mood. In enhancing motivation and encouragement, individuals' adherence and compliance to AS would be documented through this homework in reflecting their level of participation. Strategies on regular telephone follow-ups would be used to enhance individuals' motivation to complete the 8-week intervention. Depending on the couple's progress, changing or adding activities might be appropriate. In reassessment, the set of measurements as in the baseline measures would be reassessed.

2.3 Outcomes/instrument

The primary objective is to study the outcome of physical functioning of individual participants. The second objective is to study the outcome of AS on impact of caring role through assessing individual caregivers' perceived burden in care. The third objective is to study the time that needed in taking care; individuals' perception of enjoyment and achievement in their participated activities will be evaluated.

The primary outcome on impact of physical functioning is measured by the Functional Independence Measure (FIM). It is an 18-item measurement tool that explores an individual's physical, psychological, and social function [87]. The tool is used to assess a patient's level of disability as well as change in patient status in response to rehabilitation [88, 89] or medical intervention [90]. FIM is comprised of 18 items, grouped into 2 subscales—motor and cognition. The motor subscale includes eating, grooming, bathing, dressing upper body; dressing lower body, toileting, bladder management, and bowel management; transfers, bed/ chair/ wheelchair; transfers, toilet; transfers, bath/shower; walk/wheelchair; and stairs. The cognition subscale includes comprehension, expression, social interaction, problem-solving, and memory. Each item is scored on a 7-point ordinal scale, ranging from a score of 1 to a score of 7. Score 1 is total assistance with helper, 2 is maximal assistance with helper, 3 is moderate assistance with helper, 4 is minimal assistance with helper, 5 is supervision or setup with helper, 6 is modified independence with no helper, and 7 is complete independence with no helper. The higher the score, the more independent the patient is in performing the task associated with that item. The total score for the FIM motor subscale (the sum of the individual motor subscale items) will be a value between 13 and 91. The total score for the FIM cognition subscale (the sum of the individual cognition subscale items) will be a value between 5 and 35. The total score for the FIM instrument (the sum of the motor and cognition subscale scores) will be a value between 18 and 126.

The secondary outcome is to study the caregiving burden. The 22-item Chinese Zarit Burden Interview (CZBI) [91, 92] would be used to measure individuals' care burden. Scores range from 0 to 88 and higher scores indicate higher levels of burden.

The third outcome will be individuals' record of time, and activities; their perception of enjoyment and achievement will be recorded in the activity achievement worksheet (**Figure 1**) by the family caregivers. The activity achievement worksheet helps caregivers to plan activities for the week ahead that give opportunities for

Record of Activities	Sunday			Monday			Tuesday			Wednesday			Thursday			Friday			Saturday		
	Activity	E	A	Activity	E	A	Activity	E	A	Activity	E	A	Activity	E	A	Activity	E	A	Activity	E	A
0600-0800																					
0800-1000																					
1000-1200																					
1200-1400																					
1400-1600																					
1600-1800																					
1800-2000																					
2000-2200																					
2200-2400																					

Sense of enjoyment (E) and achievement (A) between 0 and 10 ('0' = no sense of enjoyment or achievement and '10' = you enjoyed the activity very much or felt a strong sense of achievement).

Figure 1.
Activity achievement worksheet.

social interaction, enjoyment, and social interaction with others. To ensure the measure of fidelity of the AS program, both experimental and control group will log their activities. With the presence of blinded assessor, these outcome measures would be administrated in baseline and after the 8-week program.

3. Results

From August 2014 to August 2018, a total of 64 community-dwelling couples, composed of older adults with CFS and their spouse caregivers, were recruited from two local day activity centers for older adults. Four participants failed to complete the consent due to language barrier. Of these couples, 30 were randomly assigned to control group and 30 were randomly allocated to experimental AS group. Two pairs of couples in control group defaulted their follow-up after the first week program. In the experimental group, one pair of couples defaulted follow-up and another one family caregiver passed away within the first two sessions of the study. Therefore, 56 pairs of couples were resulted as shown in **Figure 2**.

3.1 Baseline data

The 28 pairs of couples in the Healthcare Education group comprised 14 males and 14 females with ages ranging from 66 to 82 years (mean age = 69.25, SD = 16.32) and educational levels from 3 to 13 years (mean = 7.82, SD = 4.29). Moreover, the 28

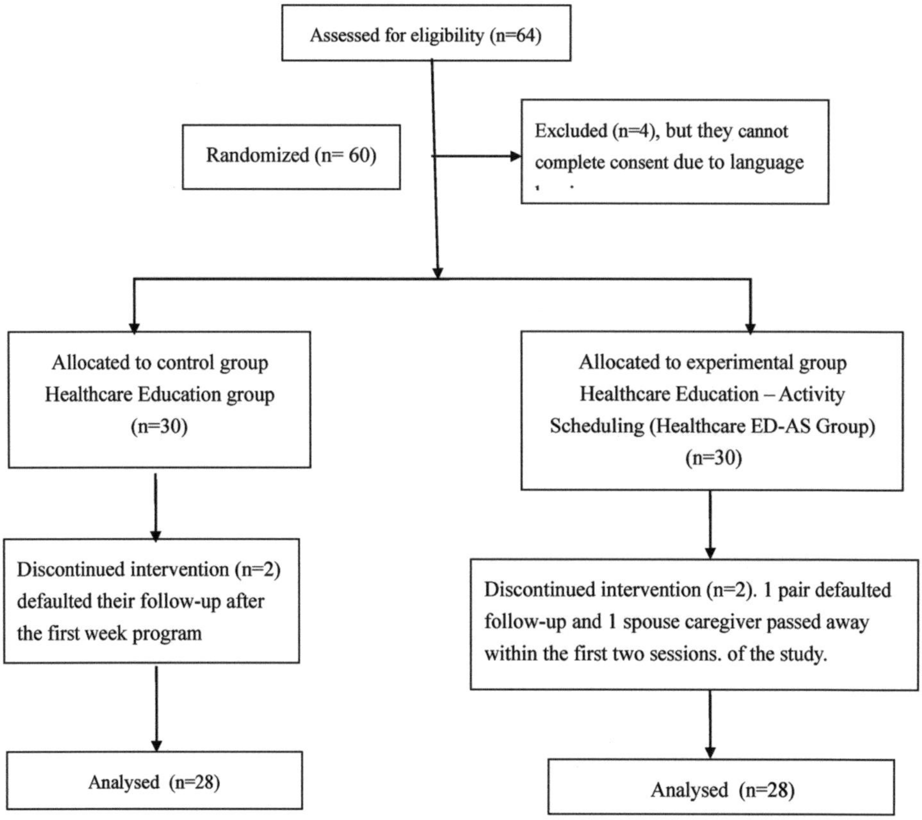

Figure 2.
Participant flow in CONSORT diagram.

participants in the Healthcare Education-Activity Scheduling (Healthcare ED-AS group) were composed of 17 males and 11 females, with ages ranging from 67 to 84 years (mean age = 70.23, SD = 12.34) and educational levels from 3.5 to 13.2 years (mean = 7.52, SD = 5.23). All recruited participants were home living. There were no significant differences between the two groups regarding age, years of education, or cognitive ability at baseline, as determined by the MoCA score (as shown in **Table 1**), and outcome measures among these groups are depicted in **Table 2**.

There were no significant differences in the baseline measurements taken for primary outcome measure on individuals' physical functioning as measured by FIM (with Cohen's d ranged from 0.02 to 0.08, $p > 0.05$). Moreover, there were no significant differences in individuals' impact of caring role (with Cohen's d ranged from 0.02 to 0.08, $p > 0.05$) and no significant difference in the amount of time spent taking care of relatives with CFS (with Cohen's d ranged from 0.03 to 0.06, $p > 0.05$).

After 8-week intervention, there were some changes in different outcome measures. For the primary outcome measure on individuals' physical functioning, paired t-test revealed a significant improvement in motor-FIM score in experimental group (with t (59) = −0.38, $p < 0.05$, with Cohen's d ranging from 0.30 to 0.44, 95% CI, 0.25 to 0.78), but not in control groups ($p > 05$).

In secondary outcome measure on the impact of caring role that was assessed using the CZBI, paired t-test revealed a significant improvement in uncertainty, subjective feeling, negative emotion, dependency, feelings of inadequacy, and total burden of care in experimental group (with t (59) = −0.38, $p < 0.05$, with Cohen's d ranging from 0.30 to 0.44, 95% CI, 0.25 to 0.78), but not in control groups ($p > 0.05$).

In the third outcome measure on caring activities, there was a significant decrease in reported caring activities on communication, use of transport, dressing, eating, and looking for appearance with Cohen's d ranging from 0.23 to 0.53.

	Healthcare Education group (n = 28)	Healthcare Education-Activity Scheduling (Healthcare ED-AS group) (n = 28)
Gender		
Older adult with CFS	Male: 14 Female: 14	Male: 17 Female: 11
Spouse caregivers	Male: 14 Female: 14	Male: 11 Female: 17
Age		
Older adult with CFS	69.25 ± 5.32	70.23 ± 5.32
Spouse caregivers	71.23 ± 4.68	71.49 ± 3.73
Education level of caregivers	From 3 to 13 years (mean = 7.82 ± 2.18)	From 3.5 to 11 years (mean = 7.79 ± 2.06)
Cognitive function (Montreal Cognitive Assessment-HK version)		
Older adults with CFS	18.16 ± 0.64	18.06 ± 0.52
Spouse caregivers	27.16 ± 0.58	28.06 ± 0.39

Table 1.
Baseline demographics and clinical characteristics for each group.

	Healthcare Education group (n = 28)	Healthcare Education-Activity Scheduling (Healthcare ED-AS group) (n = 28)	Healthcare Education group (n = 28)	Healthcare Education-Activity Scheduling (Healthcare ED-AS group) (n = 28)
	Before intervention		**After 8-week intervention**	
	Primary outcome measure			
Functional Independence Measure				
Motor-FIM	48.07 ± 1.35	48.23 ± 1.37	51.97 ± 1.57	77.47 ± 1.71
Cognitive-FIM	18.07 ± 1.36	18.19± 1.31	21.87 ± 1.82	26.53 ± 1.68
Total-FIM	66.13 ± 4.56	67.25 ± 4.35	83.96 ± 2.82	102.63 ± 1.71
	Secondary outcome measure			
Caregiver burden				
Uncertainty	8.07 ± 1.36	8.13 ± 1.31	7.97 ± 1.47	7.47 ± 1.71
Subjective feeling	22.80 ± 1.86	22.73 ± 1.74	22.70 ± 2.51	23.66 ± 2.45
Negative emotion	11.87 ± 2.22	11.70 ± 2.13	11.72 ± 3.70	10.37 ± 2.11
Dependency	9.47 ± 1.31	9.33 ± 1.30	9.48 ± 1.22	9.10 ± 1.30
Feeling of inadequacy	5.37 ± 1.40	5.40 ± 1.40	5.23 ± 1.34	4.70 ± 1.34
Total	57.56 ± 4.25	57.43 ± 4.05	57.21 ± 3.76	54.70 ± 4.46
	Secondary outcome measure			
Activity achievement worksheet				
Number of activities	11.23 ± 2.61	11.26 ± 2.32	10.84 ± 2.87	12.24 ± 1.32
Enjoyment	4.65 ± 1.79	4.71 ± 1.89	4.67 ± 1.81	6.22 ± 2.19
Achievement	4.32 ± 1.79	4.45 ± 1.85	4.26 ± 1.97	5.32 ± 1.87

Table 2.
Outcome measures for each group.

Moreover, there is a significant decrease in reported caring hour from 6.98 to 5.98 hours (with t (59) = −0.89, $p < 0.05$, Cohen's d = 0.53 with 95% CI, 0.51 to 0.68) in the experimental AS group and no significant difference in caring hours in control group from 7.02 to 7.42 hours.

In the measurement of spouse caregivers' subjective perception of enjoyment and achievement in activities they were instructed to complete an achievement worksheet. After 8-week intervention, the experimental group outperformed the control group in their number of activity participation (Cohen's d = 0.90 with 95% CI = 0.68–0.95), level of enjoyment (Cohen's d = 0.74 with 95% CI = 0.65–0.82), and sense of achievement (Cohen's d = 0.55 with 95% CI = 0.49–0.71). Moreover, in experimental group, participants reported with more physical exercise (ranging from physical exercise to more leisurely exercise, such as walking, gardening, yoga, or hiking) in their later reported figures from week 5 onward than less active physical activities (including shopping, baking, attending community events, arts and crafts, singing, and tea or lunch with friends or family) as in their earlier reported activities. Moreover, gradually increasing levels of social interaction with others were noted in experimental group than in control group. On the contrary, control group showed some more passive activities (such as reading a newspaper, watching TV, listening to the radio, looking at photo albums, and writing in a journal) throughout the period of 8-week intervention.

3.2 Within-group difference

After 8-week intervention, there were significant differences in some measures within experimental group but not in control group. For the primary outcome measure on individuals' physical functioning, paired t-test revealed a significant improvement in motor-FIM and total-FIM (with t (27) = 11.45, $p < 0.05$, with Cohen's d ranging from 0.68 to 1.64, 95% CI, 0.38 to 1.78), but not in control groups ($p > 0.05$). The secondary outcome measures on the impact of caring role. Paired t-test revealed a significant improvement in uncertainty, subjective feeling, negative emotion, feelings of inadequacy, and total burden of care in experimental group (with t (27) = −0.45, $p < 0.05$, with Cohen's d ranging from 0.43 to 0.64, 95% CI, 0.38 to 0.78), but not in control groups ($p > 0.05$).

There was significant difference in spouse caregivers' own subjective perception of enjoyment and achievement in activities within experimental group but not in control group. Following 8-week intervention, within the experimental group yielded the following results: the number of activity participation (Cohen's d = 0.52 with 95% CI = 0.48–0.65), level of enjoyment (Cohen's d = 0.74, 95% CI = 0.65–0.81), and sense of achievement (Cohen's d = 0.46 with 95% CI = 0.43–0.62).

3.3 Examine the improvement over time in intervention group

A two-group pretest-posttest ANOVA with repeated measures was conducted to compare the effect of time before and after the 8-week intervention. There was a significant effect of AS on the physical functioning of participants with CFS in experimental group, with Wilk's $\lambda = 0.72$, F (2,57) = 18.75, $p < 0.001$. Moreover, there was a significant decrease in the impact of caring role as reflected by the perceived burden of caring in the experimental group, with Wilk's $\lambda = 0.72$, F (2,97) = 18.75, $p < 0.001$. Furthermore, a study of the effect of time on caring activities for those recruited couples in AS group revealed a significant effect of AS on caring activities with Wilk's $\lambda = 0.71$, F (2,97) = 12.47, $p < 0.001$.

4. Discussion

The present study revealed that there was a positive effect of AS on improvements in activity participation in older adults with CFS. This finding echoes previous work on AS in regard to depression in older adults [82, 83]. Through this study, it became obvious that there were more activities that older adults with CFS and their spouse caregivers would like to and could participate than we expected. AS showed its advantages with the GET, CBT, and energy conservation techniques. This is very important topic as non-pharmacological interventions are needed for this hard to treat population. With the application of AS in experimental group, there was more significant improvement regarding individuals' physical functioning, as our primary outcome measure, in the experimental group. Moreover, there will be lighter perceived impact of caring role and significant reductions in uncertainty, dependency, and the feeling that caregivers were providing inadequate care. These positive changes can be partially explained by having proper channel in having more regular feedback and sharing on their caring with occupational therapists in the AS program. This channel had shown to be a strong form of support to caregivers in regard to caregiving [83, 93].

Moreover, in experimental group, AS training offered by occupational therapists focused on pleasant event scheduling and improving individuals' communication. Results indicated individuals' feelings of uncertainty and inadequacy can be greatly alleviated if they participate in activities together with the people for whom they care. The present findings echoed the effectiveness of this type of activity participation, and support had been well documented that can lower the impact of caring role in their daily lives [84, 94]. It is very important to note that not only CFS but also depression would affect people differently when it comes to their daily activities [95, 96]. It had been found that fatigue and depression had mutual interactions [97] and there can be some overlap between the two [98]. AS training showed its effectiveness in behavioral intervention for CFS. The application of AS and findings of this study can be applied to other common neuropsychological metrics such as in depression and for others with mild cognitive impairment. There were some studies that had documented its effectiveness in depression [80].

One of the most attractive assets of AS was its relatively straightforward and personalized metric in nature. With not much preparation and resources needed, it makes easy for different healthcare providers to adopt this approach in motivating our patients and their caregivers to have more activity participation. This easy-operation intervention can bring benefits to various sociodemographic levels of our society.

This study provided insights on the importance of biopsychosocial approach in the evaluation and management for CFS. Moreover, in rehabilitation, it is fundamentally important to let the participants choose activities by themselves, in order to enhance their levels of participation in the activities [99]. There were gradually increases of enjoyment and achievement and levels of social interaction noted in their reported activity achievement worksheet. It is reasonable to believe that with proper coaching and regular facilitation regarding AS by occupational therapists, activity participation in older adults with CFS can be greatly enhanced, just as it can be for other older adult populations [82, 100, 101]. This study further echoed previous well-cited studies in indicating behavioral intervention can supplement therapeutic treatment or may lead to decline in CFS symptoms [71–73, 102].

The present study relied on self-report and completion of daily activity logs in reflecting individuals' activity participation. This will limit the power of this study as social desirability bias and forgotten to complete the report would jeopardize the outcome of AS. A more standardized environment would much enhance the efficiency in building events for AS. Also, a well-cited experimental research in using neuroimaging to probe mechanisms of behavior change is needed [103]. Further resources should be solicited in making a correlation analyses with neuroimaging on justifying the effectiveness of this behavioral intervention.

Up till present, there was limited literature in showing the effectiveness of rehabilitation service for older adults with CFS. The effectiveness of AS can be further justified by conducting a study with larger group of participants and with longer-term follow-up. Regular telephone follow-ups had shown to be an effective method to maintain satisfactory compliance and adherence of caregivers; therefore, more resources should be prepared to work up closer on compliance and adherence of individuals' participation in activity and their scheduling.

Conflict of interest

The author has no relevant affiliations or financial involvement with any organization or entity with a financial interest in or financial conflict with the subject matter or materials discussed in the manuscript. This includes employment, consultancies, honoraria, stock ownership or options, expert testimony, grants or patents received or pending, or royalties. No writing assistance was utilized in the production of this manuscript.

Author details

Frank Ho-Yin Lai[1]*, Maria Uscinska[2] and Elaine Wai-hung Yan[3]

1 Department of Rehabilitation Sciences, The Hong Kong Polytechnic University, Hong Kong

2 Department of Neurosciences, Centre for Personality Disorders, University of Turin, Turin, Italy

3 Occupational Therapy Department, Kowloon Hospital, Kowloon, Hong Kong

*Address all correspondence to: frank.hy.lai@polyu.edu.hk

References

[1] Jacobson L. Hypothalamic-pituitary-adrenocortical axis: Neuropsychiatric aspects. Comprehensive Physiology. 2014;**4**(2):715-738. DOI: 10.1002/cphy.c130036

[2] Demitrack MA. Chronic fatigue syndrome: A disease of the hypothalamic-pituitary-adrenal axis? Annals of Medicine. 1994;**26**(1):1-5. DOI: 10.3109/07853899409147319

[3] Taylor RR, Kielhofner GW. An occupational therapy approach to persons with chronic fatigue syndrome: Part two, assessment and intervention. Occupational Therapy in Health Care. 2003;**17**(2):63-87. DOI: 10.1080/J003v17n02_05

[4] Papadopoulos AS, Cleare AJ. Hypothalamic-pituitary-adrenal axis dysfunction in chronic fatigue syndrome. Nature Reviews. Endocrinology. 2011;**8**(1):22-32. DOI: 10.1038/nrendo.2011.153

[5] Bock G, Whelan J. Symposium on Chronic Fatigue Syndrome. Ciba Foundation Symposium. Chichester, England/New York: Wiley; 1993

[6] Rubal E, Iwanenko W. Chronic fatigue syndrome: Is there a role for occupational therapy? Occupational Therapy in Health Care. 2004;**18**(3):33-45. DOI: 10.1080/J003v18n03_03

[7] Racciatti D, Guagnano MT, Vecchiet J, De Remigis PL, Pizzigallo E, Della Vecchia R, et al. Chronic fatigue syndrome: Circadian rhythm and hypothalamic-pituitary-adrenal (HPA) axis impairment. International Journal of Immunopathology and Pharmacology. 2001;**14**(1):11-15. DOI: 10.1177/039463200101400103

[8] Tomas C, Newton J, Watson S. A review of hypothalamic-pituitary-adrenal axis function in chronic fatigue syndrome. ISRN Neuroscience. 2013;**2013**:784520. DOI: 10.1155/2013/784520

[9] Morris G, Berk M, Puri BK. A comparison of neuroimaging abnormalities in multiple sclerosis, major depression and chronic fatigue syndrome (myalgic encephalomyelitis): Is there a common cause? Molecular Neurobiology. 2018;**55**(4):3592-3609. DOI: 10.1007/s12035-017-0598-z

[10] Cook DB, O'Connor PJ, Lange G, Steffener J. Functional neuroimaging correlates of mental fatigue induced by cognition among chronic fatigue syndrome patients and controls. NeuroImage. 2007;**36**(1):108-122. DOI: 10.1016/j.neuroimage.2007.02.033

[11] Berginstrom N, Nordstrom P, Ekman U, Eriksson J, Andersson M, Nyberg L, et al. Using functional magnetic resonance imaging to detect chronic fatigue in patients with previous traumatic brain injury: Changes linked to altered striato-thalamic-cortical functioning. The Journal of Head Trauma Rehabilitation. 2018;**33**(4):266-274. DOI: 10.1097/HTR.0000000000000340

[12] Provenzano D, Washington SD, Baraniuk JN. A machine learning approach to the differentiation of functional magnetic resonance imaging data of chronic fatigue syndrome (CFS) from a sedentary control. Frontiers in Computational Neuroscience. 2020;**14**:2. DOI: 10.3389/fncom.2020.00002

[13] Genova HM, Rajagopalan V, Deluca J, Das A, Binder A, Arjunan A, et al. Examination of cognitive fatigue in multiple sclerosis using functional magnetic resonance imaging and diffusion tensor imaging. PLOS One. 2013;**8**(11):e78811. DOI: 10.1371/journal.pone.0078811

[14] Chen Q. Neuroimaging by voxel-based morphometry: Possible approach to finding the correlation between brain structural changes and fatigue severity in patients with multiple sclerosis. American Journal of Neuroradiology (AJNR). 2011;**32**(5):880-881. DOI: 10.3174/ajnr.A2511

[15] Finkelmeyer A, He J, Maclachlan L, Watson S, Gallagher P, Newton JL, et al. Grey and white matter differences in chronic fatigue syndrome—A voxel-based morphometry study. NeuroImage: Clinical. 2018;**17**:24-30. DOI: 10.1016/j.nicl.2017.09.024

[16] Zhou Y, Lui YW. Changes in brain organization after TBI: Evidence from functional MRI findings. Neurology. 2013;**80**(20):1822-1823. DOI: 10.1212/WNL.0b013e318292a37d

[17] Zhou Y. Abnormal structural and functional hypothalamic connectivity in mild traumatic brain injury. Journal of Magnetic Resonance Imaging. 2017;**45**(4):1105-1112. DOI: 10.1002/jmri.25413

[18] Thomas K, Beyer F, Lewe G, Zhang R, Schindler S, Schönknecht P, et al. Higher body mass index is linked to altered hypothalamic microstructure. Scientific Reports. 2019;**9**(1):17373. DOI: 10.1038/s41598-019-53578-4

[19] Mittal VA, Orr JM, Pelletier A, Dean DJ, Smith A, Lunsford-Avery J. Hypothalamic-pituitary-adrenal axis dysfunction in non-clinical psychosis. Psychiatry Research. 2013;**206**(2-3):315-317. DOI: 10.1016/j.psychres.2012.12.021

[20] Atkinson HC, Leggett JD, Wood SA, Castrique ES, Kershaw YM, Lightman SL. Regulation of the hypothalamic-pituitary-adrenal axis circadian rhythm by endocannabinoids is sexually diergic. Endocrinology. 2010;**151**(8):3720-3727. DOI: 10.1210/en.2010-0101

[21] Gaab J, Huster D, Peisen R, Engert V, Heitz V, Schad T, et al. Hypothalamic-pituitary-adrenal axis reactivity in chronic fatigue syndrome and health under psychological, physiological, and pharmacological stimulation. Psychosomatic Medicine. 2002;**64**(6):951-962. DOI: 10.1097/01.psy.0000038937.67401.61

[22] Morris G, Anderson G, Maes M. Hypothalamic-pituitary-adrenal hypofunction in myalgic encephalomyelitis (ME)/chronic fatigue syndrome (CFS) as a consequence of activated immune-inflammatory and oxidative and nitrosative pathways. Molecular Neurobiology. 2017;**54**(9):6806-6819. DOI: 10.1007/s12035-016-0170-2

[23] Cevik R, Gur A, Acar S, Nas K, Sarac AJ. Hypothalamic-pituitary-gonadal axis hormones and cortisol in both menstrual phases of women with chronic fatigue syndrome and effect of depressive mood on these hormones. BMC Musculoskeletal Disorders. 2004;**5**:47. DOI: 10.1186/1471-2474-5-47

[24] Berne K. Chronic Fatigue Syndrome, Fibromyalgia and Other Invisible Illnesses: The Comprehensive Guide. Alameda, CA: Hunter House Publishers; 2002

[25] Hilgers A, Frank J. Chronic fatigue syndrome: Immune dysfunction, role of pathogens and toxic agents and neurological and cardiac changes. Wiener Medizinische Wochenschrift (1946). 1994;**144**(16):399-406

[26] Beaumont A, Burton AR, Lemon J, Bennett BK, Lloyd A, Vollmer-Conna U. Reduced cardiac vagal modulation impacts on cognitive performance in chronic fatigue syndrome. PLOS One. 2012;**7**(11):e49518. DOI: 10.1371/journal.pone.0049518

[27] Smith EM. Neuropeptides as signal molecules in common with leukocytes

and the hypothalamic-pituitary-adrenal axis. Brain, Behavior, and Immunity. 2008;**22**(1):3-14. DOI: 10.1016/j.bbi.2007.08.005

[28] Smith SM, Vale WW. The role of the hypothalamic-pituitary-adrenal axis in neuroendocrine responses to stress. Dialogues in Clinical Neuroscience. 2006;**8**(4):383-395

[29] Wojcik W, Armstrong D, Kanaan R. Is chronic fatigue syndrome a neurological condition? A survey of UK neurologists. Journal of Psychosomatic Research. 2011;**70**(6):573-574. DOI: 10.1016/j.jpsychores.2011.02.007

[30] Curtis GC, Abelson JL, Gold PW. Adrenocorticotropic hormone and cortisol responses to corticotropin-releasing hormone: Changes in panic disorder and effects of alprazolam treatment. Biological Psychiatry. 1997;**41**(1):76-85. DOI: 10.1016/s0006-3223(95)00578-1

[31] Demitrack MA, Crofford LJ. Evidence for and pathophysiologic implications of hypothalamic-pituitary-adrenal axis dysregulation in fibromyalgia and chronic fatigue syndrome. Annals of the New York Academy of Sciences. 1998;**840**:684-697. DOI: 10.1111/j.1749-6632.1998.tb09607.x

[32] Dinan TG, Majeed T, Lavelle E, Scott LV, Berti C, Behan P. Blunted serotonin-mediated activation of the hypothalamic-pituitary-adrenal axis in chronic fatigue syndrome. Psychoneuroendocrinology. 1997;**22**(4):261-267. DOI: 10.1016/s0306-4530(97)00002-4

[33] Aggarwal VR, Macfarlane GJ, Tajar A, Mulvey MR, Power A, Ray D, et al. Functioning of the hypothalamic-pituitary-adrenal and growth hormone axes in frequently unexplained disorders: Results of a population study. European Journal of Pain. 2014;**18**(3):447-454. DOI: 10.1002/j.1532-2149.2013.00413.x

[34] Altemus M, Dale JK, Michelson D, Demitrack MA, Gold PW, Straus SE. Abnormalities in response to vasopressin infusion in chronic fatigue syndrome. Psychoneuroendocrinology. 2001;**26**(2):175-188. DOI: 10.1016/s0306-4530(00)00044-5

[35] Bharadwaj S, Venkatraghavan L. Dexamethasone and hypothalamic-pituitary-adrenal axis suppression after transsphenoidal pituitary surgery. Journal of Neurosurgical Anesthesiology. 2015;**27**(2):181. DOI: 10.1097/ANA.0000000000000126

[36] Abd El-Kader SM, Al-Jiffri OH, Al-Shreef FM. Aerobic exercises alleviate symptoms of fatigue related to inflammatory cytokines in obese patients with type 2 diabetes. African Health Sciences. 2015;**15**(4):1142-1148. DOI: 10.4314/ahs.v15i4.13

[37] Patarca R. Cytokines and chronic fatigue syndrome. Annals of the New York Academy of Sciences. 2001;**933**:185-200. DOI: 10.1111/j.1749-6632.2001.tb05824.x

[38] Gur A, Cevik R, Nas K, Colpan L, Sarac S. Cortisol and hypothalamic-pituitary-gonadal axis hormones in follicular-phase women with fibromyalgia and chronic fatigue syndrome and effect of depressive symptoms on these hormones. Arthritis Research & Therapy. 2004;**6**(3):R232-R238. DOI: 10.1186/ar1163

[39] Peterson PK, Sirr SA, Grammith FC, Schenck CH, Pheley AM, Hu S, et al. Effects of mild exercise on cytokines and cerebral blood flow in chronic fatigue syndrome patients. Clinical and Diagnostic Laboratory Immunology. 1994;**1**(2):222-226

[40] Ur E, White PD, Grossman A. Hypothesis: Cytokines may be activated to cause depressive illness and chronic fatigue syndrome. European Archives of Psychiatry and Clinical Neuroscience. 1992;**241**(5):317-322. DOI: 10.1007/bf02195983

[41] Groven N, Fors EA, Iversen VC, White LR, Reitan SK. Association between cytokines and psychiatric symptoms in chronic fatigue syndrome and healthy controls. Nordic Journal of Psychiatry. 2018;**72**(8):556-560. DOI: 10.1080/08039488.2018.1493747

[42] Peterson D, Brenu EW, Gottschalk G, Ramos S, Nguyen T, Staines D, et al. Cytokines in the cerebrospinal fluids of patients with chronic fatigue syndrome/myalgic encephalomyelitis. Mediators of Inflammation. 2015;**2015**:929720. DOI: 10.1155/2015/929720

[43] Kim JW, Stewart R, Kang HJ, Bae KY, Kim SW, Shin IS, et al. Longitudinal associations between serum cytokine levels and dementia. Frontiers in Psychiatry. 2018;**9**:606. DOI: 10.3389/fpsyt.2018.00606

[44] Barroeta-Espar I, Weinstock LD, Perez-Nievas BG, Meltzer AC, Siao Tick Chong M, Amaral AC, et al. Distinct cytokine profiles in human brains resilient to Alzheimer's pathology. Neurobiology of Disease. 2019;**121**:327-337. DOI: 10.1016/j.nbd.2018.10.009

[45] Carlo-Stella N, Badulli C, De Silvestri A, Bazzichi L, Martinetti M, Lorusso L, et al. A first study of cytokine genomic polymorphisms in CFS: Positive association of TNF-857 and IFNgamma 874 rare alleles. Clinical and Experimental Rheumatology. 2006;**24**(2):179-182

[46] Moss RB, Mercandetti A, Vojdani A. TNF-alpha and chronic fatigue syndrome. Journal of Clinical Immunology. 1999;**19**(5):314-316. DOI: 10.1023/a:1020595709352

[47] Kishimoto T. Interleukin-6: discovery of a pleiotropic cytokine. Arthritis Research & Therapy. 2006;**8**(Suppl 2):S2. DOI: 10.1186/ar1916

[48] Singh-Manoux A, Dugravot A, Brunner E, Kumari M, Shipley M, Elbaz A, et al. Interleukin-6 and C-reactive protein as predictors of cognitive decline in late midlife. Neurology. 2014;**83**(6):486-493. DOI: 10.1212/WNL.0000000000000665

[49] Cullen T, Thomas AW, Webb R, Hughes MG. The relationship between interleukin-6 in saliva, venous and capillary plasma, at rest and in response to exercise. Cytokine. 2015;**71**(2):397-400. DOI: 10.1016/j.cyto.2014.10.011

[50] Leng S, Chaves P, Koenig K, Walston J. Serum interleukin-6 and hemoglobin as physiological correlates in the geriatric syndrome of frailty: A pilot study. Journal of the American Geriatrics Society. 2002;**50**(7):1268-1271. DOI: 10.1046/j.1532-5415.2002.50315.x

[51] Robson-Ansley PJ, Blannin A, Gleeson M. Elevated plasma interleukin-6 levels in trained male triathletes following an acute period of intense interval training. European Journal of Applied Physiology. 2007;**99**(4):353-360. DOI: 10.1007/s00421-006-0354-y

[52] Arnold MC, Papanicolaou DA, O'Grady JA, Lotsikas A, Dale JK, Straus SE, et al. Using an interleukin-6 challenge to evaluate neuropsychological performance in chronic fatigue syndrome. Psychological Medicine. 2002;**32**(6):1075-1089. DOI: 10.1017/s0033291702006086

[53] Ifuku M, Hossain SM, Noda M, Katafuchi T. Induction of

interleukin-1beta by activated microglia is a prerequisite for immunologically induced fatigue. The European Journal of Neuroscience. 2014;**40**(8):3253-3263. DOI: 10.1111/ejn.12668

[54] Ben-Zvi A, Vernon SD, Broderick G. Model-based therapeutic correction of hypothalamic-pituitary-adrenal axis dysfunction. PLOS Computational Biology. 2009;**5**(1):e1000273. DOI: 10.1371/journal.pcbi.1000273

[55] Giebels V, Repping-Wuts H, Bleijenberg G, Kroese JM, Stikkelbroeck N, Hermus A. Severe fatigue in patients with adrenal insufficiency: Physical, psychosocial and endocrine determinants. Journal of Endocrinological Investigation. 2014;**37**(3):293-301. DOI: 10.1007/s40618-013-0042-9

[56] Guignat L. Therapeutic patient education in adrenal insufficiency. Annales d'Endocrinologie. 2018;**79**(3):167-173. DOI: 10.1016/j.ando.2018.03.002

[57] Neu D, Mairesse O, Verbanck P, Linkowski P, Le Bon O. Non-REM sleep EEG power distribution in fatigue and sleepiness. Journal of Psychosomatic Research. 2014;**76**(4):286-291. DOI: 10.1016/j.jpsychores.2014.02.002

[58] Alves Eda S, Ackel-D'Elia C, Luz GP, Cunha TC, Carneiro G, Tufik S, et al. Does physical exercise reduce excessive daytime sleepiness by improving inflammatory profiles in obstructive sleep apnea patients? Sleep & Breathing. 2013;**17**(2):505-510. DOI: 10.1007/s11325-012-0729-8

[59] Packer TL, Sauriol A, Brouwer B. Fatigue secondary to chronic illness: Postpolio syndrome, chronic fatigue syndrome, and multiple sclerosis. Archives of Physical Medicine and Rehabilitation. 1994;**75**(10):1122-1126. DOI: 10.1016/0003-9993(94)90088-4

[60] Van Houdenhove B, Egle U, Luyten P. The role of life stress in fibromyalgia. Current Rheumatology Reports. 2005;**7**(5):365-370. DOI: 10.1007/s11926-005-0021-z

[61] Van Houdenhove B, Van Den Eede F, Luyten P. Does hypothalamic-pituitary-adrenal axis hypofunction in chronic fatigue syndrome reflect a 'crash' in the stress system? Medical Hypotheses. 2009;**72**(6):701-705. DOI: 10.1016/j.mehy.2008.11.044

[62] Monro JA, Puri BK. A molecular neurobiological approach to understanding the aetiology of chronic fatigue syndrome (myalgic encephalomyelitis or systemic exertion intolerance disease) with treatment implications. Molecular Neurobiology. 2018;**55**(9):7377-7388. DOI: 10.1007/s12035-018-0928-9

[63] Nilsson MKL, Zachrisson O, Gottfries CG, Matousek M, Peilot B, Forsmark S, et al. A randomised controlled trial of the monoaminergic stabiliser (−)-OSU6162 in treatment of myalgic encephalomyelitis/chronic fatigue syndrome. Acta Neuropsychiatrica. 2018;**30**(3):148-157. DOI: 10.1017/neu.2017.35

[64] Bjorklund G, Dadar M, Pen JJ, Chirumbolo S, Aaseth J. Chronic fatigue syndrome (CFS): Suggestions for a nutritional treatment in the therapeutic approach. Biomedicine & Pharmacotherapy. 2019;**109**:1000-1007. DOI: 10.1016/j.biopha.2018.10.076

[65] Clauw DJ. Guided graded exercise self-help as a treatment of fatigue in chronic fatigue syndrome. Lancet. 2017;**390**(10092):335-336. DOI: 10.1016/S0140-6736(17)30577-9

[66] McCully KK, Sisto SA, Natelson BH. Use of exercise for treatment of chronic fatigue syndrome. Sports Medicine. 1996;**21**(1):35-48. DOI: 10.2165/00007256-199621010-00004

[67] Pardaens K, Haagdorens L, Van Wambeke P, Van den Broeck A, Van Houdenhove B. How relevant are exercise capacity measures for evaluating treatment effects in chronic fatigue syndrome? Results from a prospective, multidisciplinary outcome study. Clinical Rehabilitation. 2006;**20**(1):56-66. DOI: 10.1191/0269215506cr914oa

[68] Wearden AJ, Morriss RK, Mullis R, Strickland PL, Pearson DJ, Appleby L, et al. Randomised, double-blind, placebo-controlled treatment trial of fluoxetine and graded exercise for chronic fatigue syndrome. The British Journal of Psychiatry. 1998;**172**:485-490. DOI: 10.1192/bjp.172.6.485

[69] Wilshire CE, Kindlon T, Courtney R, Matthees A, Tuller D, Geraghty K, et al. Rethinking the treatment of chronic fatigue syndrome-a reanalysis and evaluation of findings from a recent major trial of graded exercise and CBT. BMC Psychology. 2018;**6**(1):6. DOI: 10.1186/s40359-018-0218-3

[70] Nunez M, Fernandez-Sola J, Nunez E, Fernandez-Huerta JM, Godas-Sieso T, Gomez-Gil E. Health-related quality of life in patients with chronic fatigue syndrome: Group cognitive behavioural therapy and graded exercise versus usual treatment. A randomised controlled trial with 1 year of follow-up. Clinical Rheumatology. 2011;**30**(3):381-389. DOI: 10.1007/s10067-010-1677-y

[71] Broadbent S, Coetzee S, Beavers R. Effects of a short-term aquatic exercise intervention on symptoms and exercise capacity in individuals with chronic fatigue syndrome/myalgic encephalomyelitis: A pilot study. European Journal of Applied Physiology. 2018;**118**(9):1801-1810. DOI: 10.1007/s00421-018-3913-0

[72] Edmonds M, McGuire H, Price J. Exercise therapy for chronic fatigue syndrome. Cochrane Database of Systematic Reviews. 2004;**3**:CD003200. DOI: 10.1002/14651858.CD003200.pub2

[73] White PD, Goldsmith KA, Johnson AL, Potts L, Walwyn R, DeCesare JC, et al. Comparison of adaptive pacing therapy, cognitive behaviour therapy, graded exercise therapy, and specialist medical care for chronic fatigue syndrome (PACE): A randomised trial. Lancet. 2011;**377**(9768):823-836. DOI: 10.1016/S0140-6736(11)60096-2

[74] Gardner J, Swarbrick M, Ackerman A, Church T, Rios V, Valente L, et al. Effects of physical limitations on daily activities among adults with mental health disorders: Opportunities for nursing and occupational therapy interventions. Journal of Psychosocial Nursing and Mental Health Services. 2017;**55**(10):45-51. DOI: 10.3928/02793695-20170818-05

[75] Liu CJ, Chang WP, Chang MC. Occupational therapy interventions to improve activities of daily living for community-dwelling older adults: A systematic review. The American Journal of Occupational Therapy. 2018;**72**(4):7204190060p1-7204190060p11. DOI: 10.5014/ajot.2018.031252

[76] Lawton MP. Quality of life in Alzheimer disease. Alzheimer Disease and Associated Disorders. 1994;**8** (Suppl 3):138-150

[77] Lawton MP. Assessing quality of life in Alzheimer disease research. Alzheimer Disease and Associated Disorders. 1997;**11**(Suppl 6):91-99

[78] Lin CY, Shih PY, Ku LE. Activities of daily living function and neuropsychiatric symptoms of people with dementia and caregiver burden: The mediating role of caregiving hours. Archives of Gerontology and Geriatrics. 2019;**81**:25-30. DOI: 10.1016/j.archger.2018.11.009

[79] Au A, Gallagher-Thompson D, Wong MK, Leung J, Chan WC, Chan CC, et al. Behavioral activation for dementia caregivers: Scheduling pleasant events and enhancing communications. Clinical Interventions in Aging. 2015;**10**:611-619. DOI: 10.2147/CIA.S72348

[80] Iqbal S, Bassett M. Evaluation of perceived usefulness of activity scheduling in an inpatient depression group. Journal of Psychiatric and Mental Health Nursing. 2008;**15**(5):393-398. DOI: 10.1111/j.1365-2850.2007.01245.x

[81] Cuijpers P, van Straten A, Warmerdam L. Behavioral activation treatments of depression: A meta-analysis. Clinical Psychology Review. 2007;**27**(3):318-326. DOI: 10.1016/j.cpr.2006.11.001

[82] Riebe G, Fan MY, Unutzer J, Vannoy S. Activity scheduling as a core component of effective care management for late-life depression. International Journal of Geriatric Psychiatry. 2012;**27**(12):1298-1304. Epub 2012/03/01. DOI: 10.1002/gps.3784. PubMed PMID: 22367982; PubMed Central PMCID: PMCPMC3429703

[83] Dozeman E, van Schaik DJ, van Marwijk HW, Stek ML, Beekman AT, van der Horst HE. Feasibility and effectiveness of activity-scheduling as a guided self-help intervention for the prevention of depression and anxiety in residents in homes for the elderly: A pragmatic randomized controlled trial. International Psychogeriatrics. 2011;**23**(6):969-978. DOI: 10.1017/S1041610211000202

[84] Ruthirakuhan M, Luedke AC, Tam A, Goel A, Kurji A, Garcia A. Use of physical and intellectual activities and socialization in the management of cognitive decline of aging and in dementia: A review. Journal of Aging Research. 2012;**2012**:384875. DOI: 10.1155/2012/384875

[85] Hopko DR, Lejuez CW, LePage JP, Hopko SD, McNeil DW. A brief behavioral activation treatment for depression. A randomized pilot trial within an inpatient psychiatric hospital. Behavior Modification. 2003;**27**(4):458-469. DOI: 10.1177/0145445503255489

[86] Wong A, Xiong YY, Kwan PW, Chan AY, Lam WW, Wang K, et al. The validity, reliability and clinical utility of the Hong Kong Montreal Cognitive Assessment (HK-MoCA) in patients with cerebral small vessel disease. Dementia and Geriatric Cognitive Disorders. 2009;**28**(1):81-87. DOI: 10.1159/000232589

[87] Linacre JM, Heinemann AW, Wright BD, Granger CV, Hamilton BB. The structure and stability of the functional independence measure. Archives of Physical Medicine and Rehabilitation. 1994;**75**(2):127-132

[88] Heinemann AW, Linacre JM, Wright BD, Hamilton BB, Granger C. Relationships between impairment and physical disability as measured by the functional independence measure. Archives of Physical Medicine and Rehabilitation. 1993;**74**(6):566-573. DOI: 10.1016/0003-9993(93)90153-2

[89] Heinemann AW, Linacre JM, Wright BD, Hamilton BB, Granger C. Prediction of rehabilitation outcomes with disability measures. Archives of Physical Medicine and Rehabilitation. 1994;**75**(2):133-143

[90] Heinemann AW, Michael Linacre J, Wright BD, Hamilton BB, Granger C. Measurement characteristics of the functional independence measure. Topics in Stroke Rehabilitation. 1994;**1**(3):1-15. DOI: 10.1080/10749357.1994.11754030

[91] Ko KT, Yip PK, Liu SI, Huang CR. Chinese version of the Zarit caregiver burden interview: A validation study. The American Journal of Geriatric

Psychiatry. 2008;**16**(6):513-518. DOI: 10.1097/JGP.0b013e318167ae5b

[92] Chan TS-F, Lam LC-W, Chiu HF-K. Validation of the Chinese version of the Zarit burden interview. Hong Kong Journal of Psychiatry. 2005;**15**(1):9

[93] Burr LA, Javiad M, Jell G, Werner-Seidler A, Dunn BD. Turning lemonade into lemons: Dampening appraisals reduce positive affect and increase negative affect during positive activity scheduling. Behaviour Research and Therapy. 2017;**91**:91-101. DOI: 10.1016/j.brat.2017.01.010

[94] Teri L, Logsdon RG, Uomoto J, McCurry SM. Behavioral treatment of depression in dementia patients: A controlled clinical trial. The Journals of Gerontology. Series B, Psychological Sciences and Social Sciences. 1997;**52**(4):P159-P166

[95] Griffith JP, Zarrouf FA. A systematic review of chronic fatigue syndrome: Don't assume it's depression. Primary Care Companion to The Journal of Clinical Psychiatry. 2008;**10**(2):120-128. DOI: 10.4088/pcc.v10n0206

[96] Hulme K, Safari R, Thomas S, Mercer T, White C, Van der Linden M, et al. Fatigue interventions in long term, physical health conditions: A scoping review of systematic reviews. PLOS One. 2018;**13**(10):e0203367. DOI: 10.1371/journal.pone.0203367

[97] Fuller-Thomson E, Nimigon J. Factors associated with depression among individuals with chronic fatigue syndrome: Findings from a nationally representative survey. Family Practice. 2008;**25**(6):414-422. DOI: 10.1093/fampra/cmn064

[98] Sharpe M. Psychiatric diagnosis and chronic fatigue syndrome: Controversies and conflicts. Journal of Mental Health. 2005;**14**(3):269-276. DOI: 10.1080/09638230500136621

[99] Petruseviciene D, Surmaitiene D, Baltaduoniene D, Lendraitiene E. Effect of community-based occupational therapy on health-related quality of life and engagement in meaningful activities of women with breast cancer. Occupational Therapy International. 2018;**2018**:6798697. DOI: 10.1155/2018/6798697

[100] Mullersdorf M, Ivarsson AB. What, why, how—Creative activities in occupational therapy practice in Sweden. Occupational Therapy International. 2016;**23**(4):369-378. DOI: 10.1002/oti.1438

[101] Hunter EG, Kearney PJ. Occupational therapy interventions to improve performance of instrumental activities of daily living for community-dwelling older adults: A systematic review. The American Journal of Occupational Therapy. 2018;**72**(4):7204190050p1-7204190050p9. DOI: 10.5014/ajot.2018.031062

[102] Fulcher KY, White PD. Randomised controlled trial of graded exercise in patients with the chronic fatigue syndrome. BMJ. 1997;**314**(7095):1647-1652. DOI: 10.1136/bmj.314.7095.1647

[103] Chung T, Tittgemeyer M, Feldstein ES. Introduction to the special issue: Using neuroimaging to probe mechanisms of behavior change. NeuroImage. 2017;**151**:1-3. DOI: 10.1016/j.neuroimage.2017.01.038

Section 2

Multimodal Applications

Chapter 3

Neuroimaging Findings for Developmental Coordination Disorder (DCD) in Adults: Critical Evaluation and Future Directions

Agnieszka Anna Reid

Abstract

Approximately 75% of those diagnosed with developmental coordination disorder (DCD) exhibit motor problems in adulthood. Neuroimaging studies promise to reveal the endophenotypes of mature brain systems affected by DCD. The aim here was to review these publications. Bibliographic searches identified papers published before June 2019. Neuroimaging results revealed: functional abnormalities in the prefrontal, frontal and occipital regions, superior parietal lobe and cerebellum; structural white matter abnormalities in the corticospinal tract, internal capsule and inferior and superior longitudinal fasciculi; significantly reduced interhemispheric cortical inhibition within the primary motor cortex (hPMC); lack of increased hPMC activity during a motor imagery task and a reduced leftwards brain asymmetry for speech. These results suggest complex endophenotypes for adults with DCD (DCDAs). However, the studies have shortcomings. For instance, all relied upon small and unrepresentative samples. Gender and age were not tested systematically. The effects of many co-occurring disorders were not controlled. Most studies relied on between group comparisons, which, given the heterogeneity of DCD, may obscure the results for underrepresented cases. Overall, the young field of neuroimaging studies of DCDAs reported interesting results; however, there is an urgent need for investigations to address these shortcomings. Future research directions, including cutting-edge neuroimaging techniques and imaging genetics, are discussed.

Keywords: developmental coordination disorder, DCD, dyspraxia, adults, review, MRI, fMRI, DW-MRI, DTI, HARDI, CSD, SPECT, functional transcranial Doppler (fTCD) ultrasound, neuroimaging, individual differences, co-occurring neurodevelopmental disorders, comorbidity, genetics

1. Introduction

Developmental coordination disorder (DCD) is a common, but under-recognised neuro-developmental disorder affecting the ability to acquire motor skills, to plan motor actions and to perform actions in motor co-ordinated fashion. According to the Diagnostic and Statistical Manual of Mental Disorders 5 (DSM-5) [1], there are four diagnostic criteria for DCD. First, the impairment is characterised by significantly lower than expected (given a person's opportunity for learning and using a skill and chronological age), acquisition and execution of coordinated motor skills. Second, this motor deficit significantly interferes with the activities of everyday life, academic achievements and occupational and recreational activities. Third, DCD symptoms have their onset in early development. Fourth, deficits in motor skills are not better accounted for by intellectual or visual deficits, or neurological impairments, such as degenerative disorder, cerebral palsy, muscular dystrophy, multiple sclerosis or Parkinson's disease, which affect movement.

Different prevalence rates of DCD have been reported; however, perhaps the most reliable are the results from a large UK population study of 6990 7- to 8-year-old children [2]. This study revealed a prevalence of 1.7%. An additional 3.2% of children were identified as having 'probable DCD' by using broader cut-off criteria on tests of motor coordination and activities of daily living. Males are more often affected than females, with the male to female ratio ranging from 2:1 to 7:1 [1].

Until recently, motor-coordination difficulties in childhood were thought to be typically outgrown in adulthood. However, it is estimated that approximately 75% of those diagnosed with DCD will continue to exhibit motor problems into adulthood [3, 4]. Indeed, studies on DCDAs [5–18] demonstrate that they perform significantly worse than control participants (CPs) on various motor tasks. If one pauses for a moment and considers that the only way humans can affect the world around them is through movement (except for sweating) [19], which is crucial for communication, speech, gesture, sign-language, writing, walking, lifting, etc., it becomes obvious that difficulties with movement will cause a particularly acute deficit in a person who needs to interact with people and the surrounding world. According to the Dyspraxia Foundation [20], the range of motor deficits in DCDAs is wide, including fine motor difficulties (e.g. dressing, handwriting, sewing, putting on make-up, shaving and DIY tasks), gross motor difficulties (e.g. riding a bike, running, engaging in sports, driving a car and dancing), spatial awareness, difficulties with balance and postural control, as well as difficulties with actions which require precise timing, such as catching (e.g. a ball) and keeping up with rhythm. DCDAs also exhibit executive functioning problems in everyday life, such as difficulties organising, managing money, planning ahead and finding things in their room [21]. A glimpse of the fact that DCD adversely affects many areas of DCDA's lives is portrayed below using quotes by DCDAs.

> *'All my life I had assumed I was just "wrong" somehow. Maybe I was just stupid and lazy but was too stupid to see it. Others seemed to be better at things and I was sick of being laughed at or put up with and patronised. I hated being the one who would be slowing others down or not acting how they thought I should act. I spent much of my life just trying my best to physically catch up with other people ...' Ruth [20].*

> *'My handwriting is dreadful and it takes ages to produce anything legible. It is part of my massive problem in taking notes ...' Aileen [20].*

> *'... When I think of PE I think of being laughed at and being incredibly self-conscious for the obvious reason that PE means moving in front of other people ...' Mary [20].*

> *'I find it hard to hold my nephew comfortably for us both. I also get overwhelmed when he plays up. [...]. Spatial awareness is worse when he jumps on me and demands to be swung around etc.' Chris [20].*

Impaired motor skills in DCDAs, crucial for daily activities, have been found to be associated with lower quality of life satisfaction [22–24], difficulties with sleep, higher levels of fatigue, low self-esteem [25], depression [23, 25–27], higher anxiety [23, 26, 27], difficulties with interpersonal relationships [28], negative outcomes of education and employment [28], low participation in daily life [24] and negative consequences, but a greater ability to use coping strategies than earlier in life [29]. A need for early identification and intervention to prevent the emergence of secondary consequences was underscored [30]. Also increasing awareness of motor difficulties in DCDAs prompted researchers to start developing screening tools for DCDAs [31, 32].

Behavioural genetic studies [33, 34] reported a high heritability estimate for DCD of approximately 70%. A twin/sibling study [27] reported that approximately 0.5 of the variance in coordination difficulty in DCDAs is explained by genetic (and shared environmental) influence. Fliers et al.'s study [35] of sibling pairs with motor problems and ADHD reported a familial component of motor difficulties (comprising genetic and environmental effects) of 0.47 (rated by parents) and of 0.22 (rated by teachers). Moving on to findings from molecular genetics, a genome-wide association study (GWAS) [36] reported no significant findings. However, further analysis showed enrichment of genes for motor neuropathy and genes involved in neurite outgrowth and muscle functions. Among the highest ranked genes was *CHD6,* causing motor coordination problems in mice. These findings are certainly encouraging, but caution needs to be exercised here, because this study focused on participants with ADHD, who also exhibited motor coordination problems; therefore, they may not necessarily hold for participants with DCD. A more recent molecular genetics study [37] was the first to investigate the proportion of heritability in DCD attributed to copy number variations (CNVs—the deletion and duplication of genetic material; an increased burden of large CNVs is associated with autism, intellectual disability and schizophrenia). The results (based on 82 Canadian children with DCD, categorised into four groups—(1) pure DCD, (2) DCD + Reading Disorder, (3) DCD + ADHD, (4) DCD + ADHD + Reading Disorder and 2988 CPs) revealed an increased rate of large and rare genic CNVs and an enrichment of duplications spanning brain-expressed genes and genes previously implicated in other neurodevelopmental disorders. Some cases had a *de novo* (present for the first time) rare CNV, some inherited CNVs (64% of which came from a parent who also had a neurodevelopmental disorder). These results underscore a genetic basis for DCD and suggest that there may be shared susceptibility genes for DCD and other neurodevelopmental disorders.

DCD, similar to other neurodevelopmental disorders, poses a public health concern, but the neuropathological mechanisms underlying DCD are unknown. Analogous to other developmental disorders (e.g. developmental dyslexia and ADHD), DCD is a heterogeneous disorder [38, 39] with complex and varied manifestations. Neuroimaging studies promise new insights into this disorder. Several reviews have recently been published on neuroimaging studies on children with DCD [40–44], but not on adults. Therefore, the aim of this communication is to review neuroimaging publications involving DCDAs with the hope that they will uncover the endophenotypes of mature brain systems affected by DCD.

2. Method

Bibliographic searches of the PubMed and Web of Science databases were conducted to identify papers published before June 2019. The search terms included the following: 'adults', 'developmental coordination disorder', or 'DCD', or 'developmental dyspraxia', and either 'neuroimaging', 'ERPs', 'TMS', 'DW-MRI', 'DTI', 'fMRI', 'MRS', 'VBM', 'MRI', 'SPECT', 'MEG' and 'PET'. A total of 7 studies met the inclusion criteria (peer-reviewed studies published in English, adult participants

(≥18 years old) with DCD or well defined probable DCD who met the DSM-5 criteria for DCD, usage of at least one neuroimaging method).

2.1 Neuroimaging techniques used in the reviewed studies

For clarity, a brief description of neuroimaging techniques used in the reviewed studies is presented below.

The single-photon emission computed tomography (SPECT) imaging technique relies on the delivery of a gamma-emitting radioisotope (usually through injection to the bloodstream) into the participant. Blood flow in the capillaries of the imaged brain regions are indicated by emissions from the radionuclide. SPECT is limited by the lack of a direct measure of metabolism; however, cerebral perfusion and metabolism are closely coupled under the majority of pathologic and normal circumstances. The most common SPECT brain function measure is regional cerebral blood flow (rCBF). Two classes of radiopharmaceuticals are used in SPECT imaging: the diffusible tracers (e.g. ^{133}Xe) and the static tracers (e.g. ^{99m}Tc-ECD). The spatial and temporal resolution are better for the latter (7 mm and 20 s) than for the former (12 mm and 2 min). As SPECT uses ionising radiation, it cannot be used for experimental studies with children and for longitudinal designs, which are particularly important when studying a developmental disorder, such as DCD.

Structural magnetic resonance imaging (MRI) produces high-resolution images of the brain, with clearly distinguishable white and grey matter, fibre tracts and ventricles. It is characterised by relatively good spatial resolution such that brain structures, including subcortical structures much smaller than 1 mm, can be resolved with this method. See also Section 4.4 for more details.

Functional magnetic resonance imaging (fMRI), similar to SPECT and PET, does not directly measure neural events, but metabolic changes which are correlated with neural activity. fMRI exploits the fact that when neurons become active in a given brain area, an increase of the blood flowing to this region occurs. fMRI uses magnetic resonance imaging to measure brain activity by measuring the ratio of oxygenated to deoxygenated haemoglobin, and this value is referred to as the blood-oxygen-level-dependent (BOLD) signal. In an experimental task, brain activity is usually measured, relative to a control task. fMRI has a relatively good temporal resolution of seconds to hundreds of milliseconds and spatial resolution of 4–5 mm. See also Section 4.4 for more details.

Diffusion-weighted magnetic resonance imaging (DW-MRI) relies on the diffusion of water molecules *in vivo* to generate a contrast in magnetic resonance images. Molecular diffusion in tissues reflects interactions with membranes, macromolecules and fibres. Water molecule diffusion allows discovery of microscopic characteristics of brain tissue in a diseased or normal state. Diffusion tensor imaging (DTI) is a special type of DW-MRI. One set of questions which can be asked with DTI relates to the microstructural properties of tissues which are hypothesised to be altered in a given disease or developmental disorder. Important parameters here are the parameters reflecting the total amount of diffusion (apparent diffusion coefficient, ADC) or the fractional anisotropy (FA), defined as a scalar value between one and zero that specifies the degree of anisotropy of a diffusion process. 'One' means that diffusion takes place exclusively along one axis and is completely restricted along all other directions. 'Zero' denotes that diffusion is isotropic (unrestricted or equally restricted) in all directions. Another measure commonly used in DTI studies is mean diffusivity (MD), which is defined as a sum of the diffusivity along the principal axis (axial diffusivity) and the diffusivities in the two minor axes, divided by three. It needs to be pointed out that these measures are sensitive to many different tissue properties, such as axonal density, degree of myelination and axonal ordering. Furthermore, these measures are not specific to any one of them and this causes difficulties in interpretation of the results [45].

Although DTI is still most commonly used, it is characterised by serious limitations (for more details see Section 3.5). Therefore, recent developments have focused on the high angular resolution diffusion imaging (HARDI) data acquisition strategy. HARDI data acquisition differs only from standard DTI acquisition in which a larger number of unique diffusion-weighting gradient directions are employed, possibly utilising a larger *b*-value than required for optimal DTI acquisition. Importantly, HARDI is a technique of DW-MRI data acquisition that is necessary for methods, such as constrained spherical deconvolution (CSD) - the goal of which is to resolve the problem of the presence of multiple fibres (crossing fibres) in a single voxel (see Section 3.5, for more details).

It should be noted that structural MRI, fMRI and DW-MRI are all performed using a MRI scanner which (in contrast to PET and SPECT) does not use ionising radiation and can be used with children and in longitudinal designs.

Transcranial magnetic stimulation (TMS) is a neurophysiological technique used to stimulate the brain rather than record electrical or metabolic activity. A special coil is placed on the surface of the skull and the magnetic field passes through the skin and scalp and induces a physiological current that causes firing of the neurons. Placing a TMS coil over the hand area of the motor cortex causes (involuntary) activation of the muscles of the fingers and wrist. TMS is also used to induce temporary 'virtual lesions' by disrupting the sensory and cognitive processing of a given brain area. The consequences of the stimulation are used to shed light on the normal function of the 'lesioned' brain region, analogous to the logic of lesion studies. TMS does not use ionising radiation. The primary activation can be limited to approximately 1–1.5 cm^3; however, downstream effects also occur.

Functional transcranial Doppler (fTCD) ultrasound is a method that allows the non-invasive registration of intracranial blood flow parameters during the performance of a cognitive task. It utilises pulse-wave Doppler technology for registering blood flow velocities in the posterior, middle and anterior cerebral arteries. Analogous to other neuroimaging techniques, it is based on the close coupling between neural activation and regional cerebral blood flow changes. Because of a continuous monitoring of blood flow velocity, fTCD has better temporal resolution than fMRI.

It needs to be pointed out that the neuroimaging methods introduced above are subject to gradual improvement, with regard to their temporal and spatial resolution, as well as other characteristics. For more details on neuroimaging techniques, see [46–50].

3. Results

The following studies are included in this review: a case study involving functional and structural neuroimaging (MRI and ^{99m}Tc-ECD SPECT), four functional imaging studies (one fMRI, two TMS and one functional transcranial Doppler (fTCD) ultrasound) and two structural studies (based on DTI and HARDI with CSD)). The results were statistically significant relative to CPs. The focus is first on the case study, then on the functional imaging studies and finally on the papers on structural imaging. See also **Table 1** for the main characteristics of the reviewed studies and **Figure 1** for a summary of the imaging findings.

3.1 SPECT findings

A study using MRI and ^{99m}Tc-ECD SPECT [51] investigated a 19-year-old left-handed woman who was diagnosed with DCD at the age of 14. She was also

Study	Neuroimaging technique	Task	DCDAs[1]		CPs[2]		DCDAs and CPs	Brain areas	Findings
			N (N of males)	Mean age in years (SD)/ range	*N* (N of males)	Mean age in years (SD)/ range	Exclusion and inclusion criteria[32]		
Marien et al. [51]	^{99m}Tc-ECD SPECT Structural MRI	n/a	Case study (0)*	19	15 (8)	45–70	Diagnosed with DCD at the age of 14	31 ROI[33]	*SPECT:* Person with DCD (vs CPs): sig.[3] ↓[4] perfusion in R[5] cerebellar hemisphere and a hypoperfusion in L[6] medial prefrontal region and R occipital area *MRI:* a slight anterior/superior asymmetry of vermal fissures consistent with rostral vermis dysplasia (type 1a)
Kashuk et al. [52]	fMRI 3 T Block design (Four blocks based on difficulty)	Motor imagery	12** (5)	24.5 (7.6) 18–40	11 (6)	26.7 (5.5) 19–36	*DCDAs:* No self-reported diagnosis of ADHD, intellectual disability, autism, Asperger's Syndrome, history of neurological disease or head injury; normal cognitive and intellectual function (assumed); a standard score on MAND[7] ≤ 85 (15th percentile) on either: total score or fine or gross motor components; a score of ≥8 on the child (ADC[8]) and a score of ≥30 on total score on ADC *CPs:* a standard score on MAND ≥85 (15th percentile) on either: total score or fine, or gross motor components	Whole brain	*DCDAs (vs CPs):* sig. ↓ activation (with increasing difficulty of the task) in: L superior parietal lobe, R and L middle frontal gyrus, R and L occipital lobe/Cuneus and L cerebellar Lobule VI
He et al. [53]	Single-pulse (sp) TMS (to locate the site of the L hPMC[9]); paired-pulse (pp) TMS MEP[10]	*Intrahemispheric cortical inhibition:* CSP[11] recording, Ps[12] asked to keep voluntary muscle contraction at ~20% of MVC[13], measured by the grip force	8** (4)	23.75 (1.67) 21–32	10 (6)	26 (4.24) 21–26	*DCDAs:* No formal diagnosis of DCD, but met all the criteria according to DSM-5; ≤15th percentile for total motor composite of BOT-2[15]; ≥25 on ADC	hPMC	*DCDAs (vs CPs):* no sig. Dif.[16] on: mean SICI[17], LICI[18] and CSP Sig. ↓ interhemispheric hPMC cortical inhibition (sig. ↓ mean ISP[19])

Study	Neuroimaging technique	Task	DCDAs[1]		CPs[2]		DCDAs and CPs	Brain areas	Findings
			N (N of males)	Mean age in years (SD)/ range	*N* (N of males)	Mean age in years (SD)/ range	Exclusion and inclusion criteria[32]		
		Interhemispheric cortical inhibition: ~ 3 s before each pulse, Ps asked to perform 100% of MVC of their L hand; Ps asked to relax their hand during ITI[14]					for total score and ≥6 for the child score; *CPs:* > 20th percentile for total motor composite of the BOT-2 *Both groups:* normal intelligence (assumed); free of any self-reported medication or neurological impairments		Sig. correlation between mean ISP ratios and performance on the BOT-2 manual dexterity subtest across the groups
Hyde et al. [54]	TMS MEPs (recorded from R FDI[20] via electromyography) Stimulation latency: 50, 400 and 650 ms	Novel adaptation of HLT[21]; no instructions to Ps cueing MI[22] Ps fixated on the cross until an image of a hand appeared; they answered (using eye-movements) whether the displayed hand was L and R	8** (3)	24.29 (4.49) 20–33	21 (11)	25 (4.82) 18–36	*DCDAs:* No formal diagnosis of ADHD, dyslexia or ASD; met DSM-5 criteria for DCD; BOT-2 ≤15th percentile (except one participant's score = 16th percentile); ADC total score ≥25; ADC child score ≥6 *CPs:* age-appropriate motor abilities >20th percentile on BOT-2 *both groups:* normal intelligence (assumed); free from self-reported medication and neurological impairment	L hPMC	DCDAs who used MI (vs CPs who used MI): (1) no ↑ in corticospinal excitability; (2) a lack of change in R hand MEPs following single-pulse TMS to the L hPMC during HLT performance (relative to baseline); (3) first study to report that ↓ MI efficiency in DCDAs (vs CPs) was associated with ↓ activity of the L hPMC
Hodgson et al. [55]	fTCD[23] ultrasound	A covert word generation	12** (4)	25.33 (9.01) 18–43	12 (5)	20 (2.66) 18–28	*DCDAs:* formally diagnosed with DCD within the 10 years previous to the date of the experiment; ADC: sig. motor difficulties in childhood; scored above the diagnostic threshold on self-reported difficulties as an adult *CPs:* not specifically matched for age and gender to DCDAs	Whole brain	DCDAs (vs CPs): a sig. ↓ L lateralisation pattern for covert speech production (while no behavioural deficits for speech)

Study	Neuroimaging technique	Task	DCDAs[1]		CPs[2]		DCDAs and CPs	Brain areas	Findings
			N (N of males)	Mean age in years (SD)/ range	*N* (N of males)	Mean age in years (SD)/ range	Exclusion and inclusion criteria[32]		
							Both groups: not diagnosed with other neurological disorders; English as a first and primary language		
Williams et al. [56]	DTI	n/a	12** (6)	24.5 (7.6) 18–40	11 (5)	26.7 (5.5) 18–40	*DCDAs:* No formal DCD diagnosis; MAND score on total or component scores of ≤85 *CPs*: ≥85 on MAND score on total or component scores *Both groups:* No diagnosis of ADHD, autism or Asperger's syndrome and intellectual disability; no history of neurological disease, no head injury	ROI: R CST[24], L SLF[25], L internal capsule and R ILF[26]	*DCDAs* (vs CPs): (1) sig. ↓ FA[27] in R CST and L SLF; (2) sig. ↓ MD[28] in L internal capsule and R ILF No sig. Dif. between the groups on FA in the L internal capsule; all four ROI correlated with the total SS from the MAND; ↓ FA values in the R CST and L SLF associated with poorer motor ability ↓ MD values in the L internal capsule and R ILF also linked to poorer motor ability
Hyde et al. [57]	HARDI[29] MRI 3 T CSD[30] model and DTI model	n/a	7** (3)	23.29 (4.31) 18–46	12 (9)	26.16 (7.64) 18–46	*DCDAs:* met the DSM-5 criteria for DCD; (one participant had a previous diagnosis of DCD); scores <16th percentile for a summary of BOT-2 total; ≥25 on total score and ≥6 on child score on ADC *CPs:* > 20th percentile on BOT-2; free of self-reported medical or neurological impairment *Both groups:* No diagnosis of ADHD or similar neurodevelopmental disorder	Whole brain deterministic CSD and DTI tractography ROI: L and R CST, L and R SLF	*CSD model*: DCDAs (vs CPs): (1) sig. ↓ mean AFD[31] in the L SLF; (2) a trend for ↓ tract volume of the R SLF *DTI model:* no differences between the groups in R and L SLF microstructure *Both models:* No differences between groups in L and R CST microstructure Sig. moderate positive correlation between mean AFD of the L SLF and total BOT-2 percentile score

DOI: http://dx.doi.org/10.5772/intechopen.90400

[1]*Adults with developmental coordination disorder.*
[2]*Control participants.*
[3]*Significant.*
[4]*↓ lower/decrease and ↑ higher/increase.*
[5]*R, right.*
[6]*L, left.*
[7]*McCarron assessment of neuromuscular development.*
[8]*Adult developmental co-ordination disorders/dyspraxia checklist.*
[9]*hPMC, (human) primary motor cortex.*
[10]*Motor-evoked potential, measured by electromyography (EMG) electrodes.*
[11]*CSP, cortical silent period.*
[12]*Participants.*
[13]*Maximal voluntary contraction.*
[14]*Inter-trial intervals.*
[15]*Bruininks–Oseretsky test of motor proficiency.*
[16]*Difference/s.*
[17]*SICI, short-interval cortical inhibition.*
[18]*LICI, long-interval cortical inhibition.*
[19]*ISP, ipsilateral silent periods.*
[20]*First dorsal interosseous.*
[21]*Hand laterality task.*
[22]*Motor imagery.*
[23]*Functional transcranial Doppler (fTCD) ultrasound.*
[24]*CST, corticospinal tract.*
[25]*SLF, superior longitudinal fasciculus.*
[26]*ILF, inferior longitudinal fasciculus.*
[27]*27FA, the fractional anisotropy.*
[28]*MD, mean diffusivity.*
[29]*HARDI, high angular resolution diffusion imaging.*
[30]*CSD, constrained spherical deconvolution.*
[31]*AFD, apparent fibre density.*
[32]*Additional exclusion criteria also applied, for instance Ps with magnetic or metallic materials within their body, or suffering from claustrophobia, were not examined using the MRI scanner.*
[33]*Not fully specified.*
**Diagnosed also with developmental apraxia of speech.*
***Co-occurring developmental disorders not reported.*

Table 1.
Neuroimaging studies on DCD in adults.

diagnosed with developmental apraxia of speech. At the age of 19 years, she still had difficulties in establishing social contacts and was characterised by emotional instability and inability to maintain close relationships because of low self-esteem. Her IQ was within the normal range, but she performed better on VIQ than on PIQ (WAIS-III). She exhibited difficulties with block design (WAIS-III) and with copying the Rey-Osterrieth figure. She also had visual perception problems, distorted visual-motor integration skills and visual-motor coordination, as well as impairment of frontal planning and problem solving. There was no evidence of further cognitive deficits. Cerebellar function was tested with the Brief Ataxia Rating Scale (BARS) and revealed mild ataxia, tandem gait was not possible but was normal naturally. Her performance on the lowering of the heel was executed in a continuous axis but the movement was decomposed into several phases. Regarding the finger to nose test, oscillating movements of the hand and arm without decomposition of the movement were recorded. A few articulation errors, oral diadochokinesis and a laboured articulatory setting were noted during motor speech. The patient did not exhibit oculomotor abnormalities.

A quantified ^{99m}Tc-ECD SPECT investigation showed a significant decrease of perfusion in the right (R) cerebellar hemisphere and a hypoperfusion in the R occipital area and left (L) medial prefrontal region. Decreased perfusion in the L cerebellar hemisphere, the vermis, and the R medial prefrontal area only approached significance. Furthermore, structural MRI showed a slight anterior/superior asymmetry of vermal fissures which is in line with rostral vermis-dysplasia (type 1a). It is not clear whether this anatomical abnormality was relevant to the cerebellar functional deficit reported in SPECT examination. According to the authors, cerebellar deficiency would affect the cerebello-cerebral network involved in the execution of planned actions, visual-spatial cognition and affective regulation. On the basis of these findings, the authors concluded that the cerebellum was involved in the underlying causes of DCD.

3.2 fMRI findings

An fMRI mental rotation study by Kashuk and colleagues [52] aimed to ascertain whether adults with probable DCD (pDCDAs; not formally diagnosed with DCD, but who obtained scores on various DCD tests which indicate impairment), compared to CPs, exhibit a reduced ability when engaging in implicit motor imagery, which involves representing movements from an internal perspective, and whether they would exhibit atypical patterns of neural activation. A total of 11 adult CPs and 12 pDCDAs took part in the study. The stimulus images were pictures of R and L hands, shown so that the palm of the hand was facing the participants. They were asked to try to imagine their hand in the position of the displayed hand and decide (by pressing an appropriate button) whether they saw the R hand or L hand. Stimuli were presented in four blocks based on difficulty (Baseline (0°), Easy (40–60°), Medium (80–120°) and Hard (140–160°)). There were no significant between-group differences on response accuracy and time. Therefore, the neuroimaging results were not confounded by between-group differences on these variables. The neuroimaging results revealed significantly lower BOLD signal for increasing angle of rotation for pDCDAs than CPs in the parieto-frontal and occipito-parietal networks, including the R and L middle frontal gyrus, L superior parietal lobe, R and L occipital lobe/cuneus and cerebellar lobule VI. The authors concluded that the underactivation within the frontal, parietal and cerebellar areas may reflect deficient connectivity between areas responsible for the prospective control of movement and action planning. These results could also be interpreted as reflecting

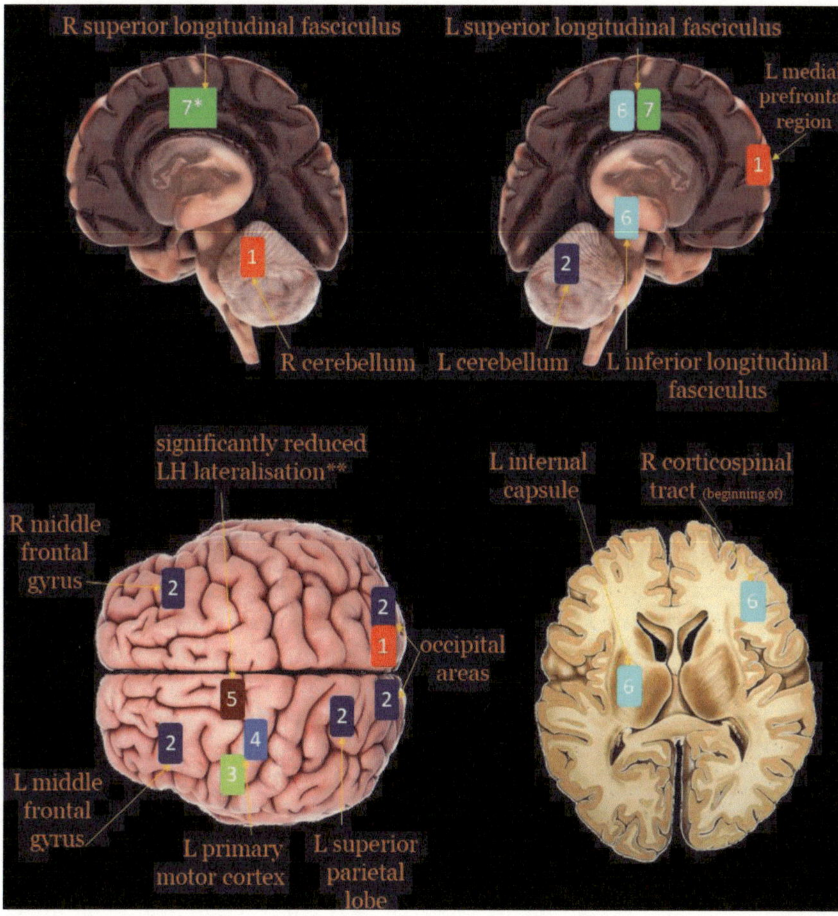

Figure 1.
Areas of non-typical brain involvement reported in neuroimaging studies of DCDAs vs. CPs displayed on the R and L medial surfaces of the brain, the brain surface viewed from above and the horizontal section of the brain. The numbers in the coloured rectangular shapes denote each neuroimaging study, as follows: 1 = Marien et al. [51], 2 = Kashuk et al. [52]; 3 = He et al. [53], 4 = Hyde et al. [54], 5 = Hodgson et al. [55], 6 = Williams et al. [56] and 7 = Hyde et al. [57]. See ***Table 1*** *for details; * denotes not a significant result, but a trend (with medium-large effect size) for decreased tract volume of the R SLF; ** denotes significantly reduced LH lateralisation in DCDAs vs. CPs.*

deficits within the underactivated areas, or even both interpretations may hold. Further studies, using different neuroimaging techniques, such as voxel-based morphometry (VBM that involves a voxel-wise comparison of the local concentration of grey matter between two groups of participants [58]), DTI (a technique which, additionally to its features described above, allows for the investigation of the anatomical structure of the axon tracts and can provide information on the between-regional anatomical connectivity between different brain areas [48]), or more sophisticated diffusion techniques, such as HARDI (with (CSD) [47]), as well as fMRI, on the same sample of pDCDAs may be able to shed further light here.

3.3 TMS findings

A study by He and colleagues [53] utilised TMS. The authors hypothesised that difficulties found in DCD, such as poor surround inhibition, compromised motor inhibition and presence of mirror movement, point to underlying problems with the regulation of inhibition within the hPMC. The aim of their study, therefore, was to test the integrity of intrahemispheric and interhemispheric cortical inhibition in the hPMC in DCDAs, as compared to CPs. A battery of single-pulse TMS and paired-pulse TMS protocols, normally employed to measure interhemispheric and intrahemispheric cortical inhibition, was used. Eight DCDAs and 10 CPs participated in the study. The results showed that, in contrast to the predictions, intrahemispheric cortical inhibition in the hPMC appeared to function normally in DCDAs. There were no group differences on mean SICI ratios (short-interval cortical inhibition—considered to activate fast-acting $GABA_A$ receptors), mean LICI ratios (long-interval cortical inhibition—presumed to activate relatively slower-acting $GABA_B$ receptors) and mean CSP ratios (cortical silent period—thought to reflect GABA receptor activity). On the other hand, congruent with the hypothesis, interhemispheric hPMC cortical inhibition was significantly reduced in DCDAs, as compared to CPs. DCDAs exhibited significantly smaller mean ISP ratios (ipsilateral silent periods—assumed to be dependent on $GABA_A$ and $GABA_B$ receptor activity), compared to CPs. Furthermore, a significant correlation between mean ISP ratios and performance on the BOT-2 manual dexterity subtest across groups, was found, indicating that reduced interhemispheric cortical inhibition in the DCDAs (and CPs) was associated with lower scores on subtests that involve bimanual coordination. It is not clear why intrahemispheric cortical inhibition in the hPMC appeared to function normally in DCDAs. A study by He and colleagues [53] was the first to provide some evidence in support for a hypothesis that regulation of GABAergic activity within the hPMC may be atypical in DCDAs. The authors argued that whereas the above results suggest that the GABAergic processes within the inactive contralateral hPMC may be preserved in DCDAs, further investigations are needed to ascertain whether modulation of these processes, flexibly, during movement, to support the suppression of unwanted movement, is possible by DCDAs, as is observed in healthy adults. Finally, as the authors focused on only the dominant (L) hemisphere, future work is needed to test cortical inhibition of the non-dominant (R) hemisphere.

A study by Hyde et al. [54] also using TMS, focused on the hPMC and aimed to test whether decreased ability in motor imagery (MI) in DCDAs, documented in behavioural studies (e.g. [59]), was associated with atypical activation in the hPMC. Single-pulse TMS was applied to the L hPMC under the assumption that changes in the contralateral hand motor-evoked potentials (MEPs) reflect activity in the hPMC. Six DCDAs and 15 CPs performed a novel adaptation of the classic hand laterality task (HLT), where participants' gaze is monitored by eye tracking and they respond visually. Single-pulse TMS was administered to the hand node of the L hPMC at three different time intervals, post stimulus presentation during the HLT. MEPs were recorded from the R first dorsal interosseous (FDI) using electromyography (a technique for registering the electrical activity produced by skeletal muscles). The results showed that 75% of DCDAs and 71% of CPs engaged in MI during the HLT and there was no significant difference between the groups; only these participants were included in the analysis because modulation of the hPMC during HLT performance is considered as being dependent on the MI strategy. MI users with DCD were significantly less efficient than MI using CPs. In contrast to CPs, no evidence of increased hPMC activity during MI was detected in DCDAs. The authors concluded that their data were consistent with the hypothesis that inefficient MI in DCDAs may be due to underactivation of the hPMC. It would be of importance to investigate the structural and functional characteristics of the hPMC in DCD using structural MRI (with VBM) and functional imaging methods, such as fMRI and MEG in the same sample of DCDAs. Furthermore, as pointed out by the authors, future work also needs to address the role of downstream mechanisms in the deficient activity in the hPMC in DCDAs.

3.4 fTCD ultrasound findings

A study by Hodgson and colleagues [55] used fTCD ultrasound. Given research evidence suggesting that the typical pattern of hemispheric specialisation is altered in individuals with neurodevelopmental disorders, such as SLI and dyslexia, the authors assessed whether DCDAs exhibit reduced L hemisphere lateralisation for speech production compared to CPs [55]. Twelve DCDAs and 12 CPs performed a covert word generation task while undergoing fTCD. All DCDAs had been diagnosed with DCD within the 10 years previous to the date of experimental examination. The results showed that DCDAs exhibited a significantly reduced L lateralisation pattern for the speech production task, relative to CPs, with no behavioural deficits for speech. Therefore, the fTCD results could not have been confounded by behavioural speech deficits. Following the results of a study which reported that CPs with the *KIAA0319/TTRAP/THEM2* gene variants [60] (identified as increasing the risk of developmental dyslexia) exhibited a reduced L hemispheric asymmetry of the superior temporal sulcus (during a reading task), it may be possible in future research to link specific gene variants to the significantly reduced L lateralisation pattern for speech production reported in DCDAs [55], using an imaging genetic approach.

3.5 DW-MRI findings

A DTI study by Williams and colleagues [56] investigated whether white matter microstructure alterations reported in children with DCD [61–63] were also present in pDCDAs. Twelve pDCDAs and 11 CPs underwent DTI. The results revealed that the pDCDAs (in comparison with CPs) exhibited significantly lower FA in the superior longitudinal fasciculus (SLF) and the corticospinal tract (CST). Furthermore, pDCDAs (in comparison with CPs) had lower MD in the inferior longitudinal fasciculus (ILF) and internal capsule. These results suggest that there were significant (most likely persistent throughout the life span), neurobiological alterations in the microstructural properties of the white matter in these white-matter structures between pDCDAs and CPs. The result of reduced FA in the SLF is congruent with the findings reported for children by Langevin and colleagues [62]. In contrast, the finding of lower FA in the CST tract does not replicate previous findings for children [63]. However, it has to be born in mind that given the considerable heterogeneity of DCD, the results are not directly comparable because these studies tested different individuals who also markedly differed in age range (18–40 years [56] and 8–12 years [63]). As DTI (or (HARDI)) with (CSD) is not an invasive method, and does not use ionising radiation, it would be desirable to clarify these differences in a longitudinal study which starts in childhood and continues into adulthood.

All studies on white matter organisation in DCD participants relied on DTI. However, as DTI uses a single tensor to estimate fibre orientation within a voxel, it is only able to resolve a single fibre orientation per voxel and cannot represent multiple fibres in a single voxel (the 'crossing fibre' problem). Because fibres cross in up to 90% of white matter voxels [64], DTI technique is prone to providing incorrect reconstructions or spurious white matter tracts and therefore caution is needed when interpreting DTI results [65]. Bearing in mind this criticism, Hyde and colleagues [57] reported a pilot study, exploring CSD—a method robust to the issue of 'crossing fibres' that calculates apparent fibre density (AFD)—a metric of intra-axonal volume fraction [66], with higher values likely indicating greater axon diameter or local axon count [67]. The white matter tissue organisation of the sensorimotor tracts in DCDAs was examined using CSD. Seven DCDAs and 12 CPs underwent HARDI. The R and L CST and SLF were delineated and all tracts were then generated using both CSD and DTI tractography. DCDAs demonstrated significantly decreased mean AFD in the L SLF relative to CPs and a trend for decreased tract volume of the R SLF, on the basis of the CSD model. When using the DTI model, no between group differences were found in SLF microstructure. Furthermore, there were no between group differences in the bilateral CST microstructure regardless of the diffusion model. Finally, a significant moderate positive correlation between mean AFD of the L SLF and total BOT-2 percentile score was found, revealing a relationship between motor performance and diffusion metrics. The authors interpreted the results as being consistent with the hypothesis according to which the motor impairment observable in DCD may be due to white matter abnormalities in sensorimotor tracts, especially in the SLF. More specifically, they emphasised that their results suggest that DCDAs (in comparison to CPs) are characterised by decreased axon diameter or decreased axon count in the L SLF and in R SLF (a non-significant trend). As the authors pointed out, this is of interest because smaller axonal diameter has been linked to slower axonal conduction. The results from Hyde and colleagues' study based on CSD seem very promising. However, the authors did not replicate the CST abnormality found in the study reported by Williams and colleagues [56], and relied on a small sample of participants; therefore, the results of Hyde and colleagues' study need to be replicated with a larger sample of DCDAs.

3.6 Summary and critique

Summarising, the neuroimaging results revealed functional abnormalities in the R cerebellar hemisphere, L medial prefrontal hemisphere and R occipital region [51], L superior parietal lobe, bilateral middle frontal gyrus, bilateral occipital lobe/cuneus and L cerebellar Lobule VI [52]. Structural white matter abnormalities were found in the R CST and L SLF, L internal capsule and R ILF [56] and in the L SLF with a trend for abnormality in the R SLF, with no abnormality in the microstructure of the CST [57]. Furthermore, DCDAs exhibited significantly reduced interhemispheric cortical inhibition within the hPMC [53], lack of evidence of increased hPMC activity during a motor imagery task [54] and a reduced leftwards brain asymmetry for speech [55]. These results suggest that, similar to neuroimaging findings on children with DCD [40], DCD manifests as a complex neurodevelopmental disorder in DCDAs. DCDAs' unresolved motor problems from childhood persist into adulthood and are associated with functional and structural brain abnormalities.

However, a majority of reviewed studies have shortcomings. First, most of the studies relied for convenience on small, unrepresentative and underpowered samples which are problematic, especially when dealing with a heterogeneous disorder, such as DCD; Second, some studies relied on adults with probable DCD, rather than adults with diagnosed DCD, and this may have added to the heterogeneity across the samples. It should be mentioned here that according to the International Clinical Practice Recommendations for DCD [68], presently there are no explicit diagnostic criteria for DCD for adults. DSM-5 mentions adults and it has been interpreted that the same criteria as for children, with small adaptations, may be used for adults [68]. Furthermore, there are no standardised assessments for DCDAs, except for BOT-2 (norms up to 21 years, but only for USA and Germany) and MAND (norms for 18–35 years), but they are more than 20 years old. These factors make diagnosing DCD in adults difficult. Because the age of some adults with probable DCD, included in the reviewed studies, lies outside the norms for BOT-2 and MAND, the results must be interpreted with caution. Third, gender and age were not tested systematically. These variables are important, because DCD seems to be a disorder characterised by gender bias and important gender differences in DCD were reported by, for instance, studies on environmental factors (see Section 4.5 below); also neuroimaging studies on other developmental disorders, e.g. dyslexia have revealed gender-specific grey matter volume differences [69]. Furthermore, crucial maturation processes take place in brain development in adolescence and adulthood [70, 71]; therefore, age ranges that include young adults and middle-aged adults, reported in more than a half of the reviewed studies, are not advisable cf. [40]. Fourth, most studies have potential confounds because DCD co-occurs with other neurodevelopmental disorders, such as dyslexia and ADHD and many others (for more details see the Section 4.1 below), most of which were not controlled for in the reviewed studies. Fifth, DCD is a heterogeneous disorder; hence, reliance on between-group comparisons might obscure the results for underrepresented cases. Sixth, prenatal and perinatal history (shown to impact neurological findings) was not reported in any of the reviewed studies. Seventh, the studies usually only provide a small number of DCD measures; however, it would be desirable that more extensive testing of motor abilities were included, giving an in-depth description of the nature and severity of the motor difficulties. As there is now growing evidence of cerebellar deficit in DCD, it would also be advisable to test the cerebellar function behaviourally in participants with DCD. Finally, as DCD is a developmental disorder, longitudinal studies are needed to understand the deficits in this disorder—it is likely that manifestations of deficits in DCD will differ in different developmental stages.

Overall, although the neuroimaging studies on DCDAs reviewed above, reported interesting results, the small number of studies, small unrepresentative samples and limited number of neuroimaging techniques indicate that, in comparison to neuroimaging studies on other developmental disorders, neuroimaging in DCDAs is a very young field. Therefore, there is an urgent need for further neuroimaging studies on DCD which would address the above-mentioned shortcomings. Future directions for DCD research, including cutting-edge neuroimaging techniques and imaging genetics, are discussed below.

4. Future directions

4.1 Studies on the underlying causes of DCD

Within the field of DCD research, there is an urgent need for studies which focus on investigating the underlying causes of DCD. The current research indicates that the co-occurrence of neurodevelopmental disorders is most likely more common than cases of 'pure' disorders [72] with up to 70% of children meeting the criteria for at least one other neurodevelopmental disorder [73]. Motor deficits have been associated with a considerable number of developmental disorders, although quite often it was considered to be part of a given disorder, rather than a part of possibly co-occurring DCD [74]. There is growing evidence that DCD co-occurs with many other disorders, such as ADHD (the most frequent co-occurring disorder, in approximately 50% of cases), dyslexia, dysgraphia, speech and language disorder, autism spectrum disorder, visual perception deficit, joint hypermobility syndrome and disruptive and emotional behavioural problems [1]. Furthermore, co-occurrence with other disorders such as specific language impairment (SLI) [75], developmental apraxia of speech [51] and arithmetic and working memory difficulties [76] was also noted. At present the relationship between DCD and co-occurring disorders is not clear. It should be emphasised here that although efforts were made to control the effects of some co-occurring disorders (e.g. ADHD), the effects of many other potentially co-occurring disorders were not controlled for in the reviewed studies. Therefore, there is an urgent need for future research on the underlying causes of DCD to control for the effects of these either by the exclusion of cases with such disorders or by collecting appropriate data from cases with co-occurring disorders to be entered as covariates in analyses. Otherwise the results would be confounded by the effect of co-occurring developmental disorders and no claims could be made with regard to the effects of DCD. For a similar argument regarding research on developmental dyslexia see [77, 78].

An important issue in investigating the underlying causes of DCD is to use a robust theoretical framework. A single deficit model has been dominant for many years in the research on neurodevelopmental disorders. For instance, according to the internal modelling deficit (IMD) hypothesis [79], the movement difficulties in DCD are due to a deficit in the ability to engage predictive control during planning and executing movements. This is concluded from the evidence on participants with DCD (DCDPs) who, in comparison to CPs, exhibit deficient motor imagery, a smaller amount of anticipatory postural adjustment when initiating movement and slower adjustments to target perturbations during the action of reaching [80]. However, a single deficit model, although parsimonious and relatively easy to test, has limitations. For instance, as underscored by Wilson and colleagues [80], IMD hypothesis is supported, among other results, by behavioural data on effector systems, but deficits were stronger on tasks that involved higher complexity or required more endpoint precision. These indicate that some other deficits may be involved. Furthermore, the results from neuroimaging studies reported that abnormalities in brain function and structure are also present in areas that do not belong to IMD/MNS (mirror neuron system) networks; for instance, in children with DCD (compared to CPs), significantly lower BOLD in L superior frontal and lingual gyri was reported [81, 82]. Therefore, it may be a fruitful way forward to consider a multiple deficit model (MDM), similar for instance to that proposed for developmental dyslexia [83]. According to MDM, more than one deficit is necessary to cause a given developmental disorder, such as DCD. In contrast to a single deficit model, MDM can account for any more frequent than chance co-occurrence of the neurodevelopmental disorder with another neurodevelopmental disorder.

Another model that needs to be considered here is the recently proposed hybrid (multicomponent) model of motor skill development based on advances in cognitive neuroscience and ecological systems theory [80]. It consists of three components: individual, task and environment. The individual level is most complex and consists of motor abilities, motor and cognitive processes and biological maturation and genetics. Importantly, motor performance emerges from the interaction of these three components (for more details see [80]). This model may prove particularly valuable for longitudinal studies of DCD. Finally, the neural systems hypothesis (NSH) [84] may also prove to be a useful framework for further DCD research. According to this hypothesis, research on developmental disorders can be unified by the claim that their underlying cause is a deficient procedural learning system. The main underlying cause of DCD is classified by NSH as a motor-cortico-striatal deficit. Participants with DCD, who also suffer from verbal dyspraxia (like the person in the case study reported above [51]), might also be classified as having language-cortico-striatal difficulties. It could not be stressed more that discovering the underlying causes of DCD is of vital importance, not only for gaining insight into this neurodevelopmental disorder but also for designing appropriate interventions.

4.2 Neuroimaging studies using longitudinal designs

The reviewed studies investigated DCD in adults. Such studies are undoubtedly important because through them an insight into the neural correlates of DCD in a mature system is gained. Furthermore, focus on adults with DCD allows one to bypass a potential problem of the presence of the sub-group of children with DCD who 'grow out' of their motor difficulties [56]. However, it is possible that the adult neural system may have been partially or greatly altered due to compensatory mechanisms, as a reaction to brain abnormalities. Furthermore, providing that motor skills (gross and fine) are learned over a relatively protracted period of time, it is likely that brain-based findings are going to be dynamic and change over time. Therefore, as well as continuing research on adults with DCD, there is an urgent need to develop longitudinal neuroimaging studies, starting with infants from families at risk of DCD, so that the developmental trajectory of deficits in DCD can be tracked over time.

4.3 Focus on individual differences in DCDAs

The issue of individual differences is crucial in studying and understanding heterogeneous developmental disorders; however, it is usually (with few exceptions, e.g. [77, 78]) neglected. As stated earlier in this chapter, DCD is a heterogeneous disorder, hence reliance on between-group comparisons (with a group consisting of participants with DCD (DCDPs) being most likely heterogeneous) might obscure the results for underrepresented or rarer cases. Furthermore, the proportion of individuals with DCD having a different profile in a given sample can vary across studies, resulting in non-congruent results. Therefore, a promising way forward in DCD research would be to carry out multiple case studies that focus on individual differences. Another fruitful and more powerful direction would be to compile an extensive test battery to identify sub-groups of DCDPs, as homogeneous as possible, and these in turn may then be compared on dependent variables to CPs or to each other.

4.4 Extending the types of imaging tools used in DCD research

The reviewed studies used structural MRI, SPECT, fMRI, TMS, functional transcranial Doppler (fTCD) ultrasound, DTI and HARDI. This is only a subset of currently available neuroimaging tools, and usage of additional neuroimaging techniques may shed new light on the DCD endophenotype. Given that interesting findings from magnetic resonance spectroscopy (MRS) have been obtained for developmental dyslexia [85] and ADHD [86], it seems promising to use this technique to investigate DCDPs. MRS is the only research tool that allows a non-invasive *in vivo* assessment of neurochemical aspects of a given disorder without using ionising radiation. It obtains a measure of the quality of brain tissues and detects concentrations of specific neuro-metabolites *in vivo*, such as: *N*-acetylaspartate (NAA), *N*-acetylaspartate plus *N*-acetyl-aspartyl-glutamate (tNAA), choline (Cho), creatine (Cr), creatine plus phosphocreatine (Cr + PCr), GABA, glutamate (Glu), glutamine (Gln), glutamate plus glutamine (Glx), myo-inositol (mI), myo-inositol-containing compounds (Ino), freely mobile membrane phospholipid precursors (free-PME) and freely mobile membrane phospholipid breakdown products (free-PDE). For more details on MRS, see [87].

Findings from investigations using DTI [56] and HARDI (with CSD model) [57] on DCDAs and children with DCD [61–63] that suggest white matter abnormalities and results from an MRS study which revealed that heightened levels of choline are associated with abnormalities in white matter [88], prompt the important empirical question of whether both deficits can be found with HARDI and MRS in the same sample of DCDPs. Furthermore, findings by He et al. [53], discussed above, provide the first evidence in support of a hypothesis that regulation of GABAergic activity within the hPMC may be atypical in DCDAs. Therefore, it would be desirable to explore concentrations of GABA in the hPMC in DCDAs using MRS.

Participants with DCD exhibit poor sensorimotor coordination, which among other processes, involves precise timing and using feedback to respond to changes in the environment [89]. Therefore, neuroimaging techniques with good temporal resolution, such as EEG and MEG combined with rigorous scientific experimental designs, may be able to shed new light on the endophenotypes of DCD. Such investigations look even more promising due to recent developments in MEG where new, advanced pre-processing techniques enable decomposition of the signal into components with their origin inside and outside the head. This increases the signal-to-noise ratio by approximately 100%, enabling therefore even one-trial measurements with the standard MEG systems. Furthermore, a considerable increase of MEG signal-to-noise ratio is now possible thanks to optically pumped magnetometers that allow MEG sensors to get closer to the head [90].

There are emerging findings that neurodevelopmental disorders are associated with structural and functional abnormality within the default mode network (DMN). DMN is a large-scale brain network of interacting brain areas characterised by highly correlated activity with each other. It is activated when individuals focus on internal tasks such as retrieving memories, daydreaming and imagining the future. It is distinct from other networks in the brain. Evidence points to disruptions in the DMN of people with neurodevelopmental disorders, including ASD [91, 92] and ADHD [92]. Therefore, it would be advisable to investigate whether this is also the case for individuals with DCD. DMN seems well suited for usage with participants with neurodevelopmental disorders, such as DCD, because it can be measured with effortless and short resting-state scans and can be performed with any population, including children, and may be used in studies with longitudinal designs.

DMN is one of a number of resting-state conditions identified in the brain and researched. Another line of investigation here is whole-brain resting-state functional connectivity (rsfMRI), a technique used to measure intrinsically organised patterns of spontaneous signal fluctuations across the whole brain. Interestingly, a recent study [93] applied a multivariate data-driven approach (where diagnostic categories were not used) to discover latent components linking a large set of cognitive, clinical and personality measures to whole-brain resting-state functional connectivity patterns across CPs and participants with ADHD, schizophrenia, schizoaffective disorder or bipolar disorder. Three latent components—cognitive dysfunction, general psychopathology and impulsivity were discovered. Remarkably, every component was characterised by connectivity alterations within the somatosensory-motor network and in its connections to the cortical executive and subcortical networks. These results identify three latent components as plausible cross-diagnostic phenotypes, which account for comorbidity across disorders. Interestingly, alterations within the somatosensory-motor network is of importance to all the cross-diagnostic phenotypes. Such an approach should also be fruitful in the investigation of DCD and the co-occurring disorders.

There is growing evidence that DCDPs exhibit difficulties in interpersonal interactions [20, 51]. Currently it is not clear whether this is due to pure DCD or to co-occurrence with ADHD and/or ASD. Such difficulties can lead to social isolation and later to depression. Until recently, there was no easy way to study social interaction with neuroimaging. However, in 2009, a 'two-person neuroscience' (2PN), an approach to study the physiological basis of social interaction, was proposed [94]. One of the main experimental goals of 2PN was to differentiate reactive vs. interactive states of human social interaction by measuring simultaneously brain signals from two participants. As natural social interaction involves exchange of information between the participants at time intervals shorter than 100 ms, brain imaging methods with good temporal resolution, such as MEG or EEG are indispensable. Recently, a first set-up for simultaneous MEG-to-MEG recordings was built [95]. The main strength of MEG over EEG in the simultaneous set up recordings is that the sources of the signals (e.g. brain rhythms modulation) can be identified with higher accuracy. Instead of estimating connectivity between regions of a given participant's brain, hyperconnectivity, a measure of functional connectivity between the brains of two participants, can be calculated. With data obtained from two brains in a simultaneous recording, one can investigate the correlations between the two sets of brain signals without explicit reference to the external events [95]. 2PN certainly therefore seems to offer a promising way forward for investigating participants with DCD where interpersonal relationships are affected. However, it should be emphasised here that these are still early days and the data analysis of 2PN is challenging.

Finally, advances in MRI and fMRI, such as multiband fMRI [96] and high-field MRI [97], promise to increase the spatial and or temporal resolution of these neuroimaging methods, ensuring that they will continually serve as powerful neuroimaging tools for investigating the structure and function of the brain in DCD.

Given the heterogeneity of DCD, it is unlikely that one biomarker for this disorder will be sufficient. Therefore, studies that employ more than one neuroimaging technique, for instance, VBM, HARDI (with CSD model) and fMRI with the same sample of participants with DCD, as mentioned in the context of Kashuk et al.'s [52] study, are urgently needed.

In summary, the advances discussed above offer many new possibilities in DCD neuroimaging research. DCD endophenotypes can be investigated with higher spatial and temporal resolution, their DMN and resting-state functional connectivity can be tested, the concentration of metabolites, especially GABA can be determined and utilising 2PN with simultaneous MEG-to-MEG recordings can shed new light on the interacting DCD brain. Finally, using different neuroimaging techniques with the same sample of DCDPs will allow for asking more precise questions. All of these will increase the chances of elucidating the underlying causes of DCD and reliable biomarkers for DCD.

4.5 Environmental factors in DCD

DCD is a multifactorial disorder in which genetic factors and environmental factors as well as gene x environment interactions play a role. As described above, some efforts were made to discover the genetic factors involved in DCD. The research on the environmental factors that influence DCD is limited. The importance of environmental factors was underscored in DSM-V by introducing the new exclusion criterion for DCD, namely the lack of opportunity for skill learning and use. So far, the following environmental factors have been identified as increasing the risk of developing DCD: lower birthweight (less than 2500 g), being born before 37 weeks of gestation and lower socioeconomic status [2], being born pre-term, being small for gestational age or being 15 months of age or more at walking attainment [98], prenatal exposure to alcohol [1], Caesarean section, maternal pre-eclampsia and low income [99]. Interestingly, gender differences have been reported. Lower than optimal birthweight was associated with poorer motor outcomes in males, whereas, smoking during early pregnancy and stress during later pregnancy were linked to poorer motor development in females [99]. Future studies need to keep testing and refining the knowledge of environmental risk factors in DCD. The research on the underlying causes of DCD needs to collect data on risk factors for DCD and enter them into the analyses to reduce the number of confounds.

4.6 Genetic research

Neuroimaging studies provide descriptions of endophenotypes, but do not offer an explanation as to what is the underlying cause of a given disorder. For this, researchers need to investigate the genetic basis of DCD. In comparison to research on other developmental disorders, genetic research on DCD is lagging behind. Nevertheless, some promising strides have been published, as described in the introduction. An ultimate goal for future genetic research is to ascertain which variants of which genes are risk factors for developing DCD. One way forward here would be to develop high quality GWAS with large, representative samples. The assumption of GWAS is that common variants underlie common disorders and, therefore, they focus on sampling sites of known common genetic variation. GWAS rely on 'arrays' and they only genotype the pre-defined sites of variation and do not sequence every base. Therefore, GWAS cannot be used for searching for rare or new variants within a genome [100]. As it is likely that both common and rare genetic variations contribute to disorder risk in DCD, genome sequencing technologies would be beneficial. This is because they record both common and rare variants, as well as CNVs. However, it has to be born in mind that this technology remains relatively expensive and, as large samples are necessary, the collection of participants with DCD may need to involve international collaboration.

It is very difficult to ascertain the functional impact of genetic variation; however, mouse models have the potential to make an impact on the understanding of the underlying causes of neurodevelopmental disorders, such as DCD. Initial efforts involving mouse models seem promising [101–103]. More recently, in research in progress, the authors [104] used recombinant inbred lines of mice, 12 BXD strains and parental strains C57BL/6J and DBA/2J to investigate DCD. BXD27 mice, characterised by smaller cerebellar volume, showed motor impairments across different skills; the researchers also plan to collect data from brain imaging, so that more light can be shed on the basis of poor motor learning and coordination in BXD27 mice.

The significance of discovering the variants of genes which are genetic risk factors for DCD cannot be emphasised strongly enough. This would open the door to many further investigations, such as imaging genetics, which provides a bridge between the brain and behaviour. For instance, imaging genetics will allow for linking gene variants to the functional and structural abnormalities of grey matter and structural abnormalities of white matter. Such research is more advanced regarding other developmental disorders, e.g. ADHD and developmental dyslexia [78]. Finally, it needs to be underscored that the biological complexity of DCD cannot be disregarded and genome-wide measurements, together with investigations of individual genes and pathways, are crucial in ascertaining the underlying mechanisms of neurodevelopmental disorders, such as DCD [105]. See also the Sections 4.7 and 4.8 below.

4.7 Neuroimaging intergenerational transmission of brain circuitry

Intergenerational neuroimaging is a relatively recent approach that uses neuroimaging to test the relationship of neural and cognitive phenotypes between parents and their children. It is based on the fact that there is a transfer of traits from parents to offspring which consists of both non-genetic and genetic influences. The impact of prenatal effects (e.g. parent nutrition and *in-utero* environment), rearing effects and other environmental factors could cause epigenetic changes (changes in gene function in the absence of gene sequence changes) or behavioural changes in the children, which are transmitted intergenerationally [106]. Intergenerational neuroimaging may be a promising way forward in clarifying the ontogeny of complex neurodevelopmental disorders, such as DCD. One way of disentangling inherited factors from pre- and postnatal influences is by utilising the potential of natural cross-fostering designs that take advantage of different types of *in vitro* fertilisation (homologous surrogacy (mother is egg donor and birth mother), donor egg pregnancy (mother is not egg donor but is birth mother) or heterologous surrogacy (mother is egg donor but not birth mother)) [106]. Such designs hold promise to address many crucial questions in DCD research. For instance, what are the intergenerational effects on the brain structure and function, including those involved in coordinated movement? What is the impact of gender-specific effects at the prenatal stage (particularly important as DCD is more prevalent in males than females [1]), including the effects of prenatal testosterone levels on brain development, and gender-specific transmission patterns [107, 108] in movement-related brain circuits in newborns.

4.8 Integrative neuroimaging

As discussed above, an inherent difficulty in the research on neurodevelopmental disorders is their heterogeneity. Another stumbling block here is the fact that neurodevelopmental disorders are characterised by pleiotropy [105]. These are some of the most heritable disorders, but simultaneously they also are extremely complex genetically. For instance, a dosage of CNV increases one's risk for multiple diagnosis and conversely, given a single diagnosis of developmental disorder, one can reach it from multiple genetic starting points. Therefore, if one wants to find a biomarker, for instance dyslexia, one immediately carries together a group of different genetic conditions, as defined by their genotype. Because of these obstacles, an alternative approach has been proposed [109–111], namely trying to first understand the biology of neurodevelopmental disorders with genetically defined groups, such as those with sex chromosome aneuploidy (SCA) syndrome. This strategy can be helpful because the genetic makeups in SCA syndrome are known. It should be emphasised here that having additional sex chromosomes increases the risk for diverse neurodevelopmental disorders, especially those that impact social function and interaction, as well as language. The SCA model may be used to understand how CNV can cause changes in brain systems relevant to neurodevelopmental disorders. Therefore, the SCA syndrome has become the genetically defined risk model for neurodevelopmental disorders [112].

Taking advantage of the growing number of publicly available molecular and cellular maps available in the standard neuroimaging atlas space, such as the Allen Brain Atlas [113] and BigBrain [114] and structural MRI, it has been reported that patients with increasing X or Y chromosome dosage tend to have disproportionally reduced size of cortical brain surface area, such as L posterior insula, L and R anterior cingulate, L gyrus rectus, R anterior cingulate and R posterior orbital gyrus. These patients also exhibit reduced size of cortical thickness of L and R superior temporal sulcus/medium temporal gyrus, increased cortical thickness of L medial prefrontal cortex, L and R parahippocampal cortex and R orbitofrontal cortex, as well as increased cortical surface area of L and R precuneus [110]. Furthermore, meta-analysis of brain activation patterns across more than 5000 functional neuroimaging publications has revealed that these areas are involved in the detection and processing of biological motion, language, autobiographical memory, reward, affect and interoception [110]. These cognitive domains seem relevant to social functioning and language. It is important to mention that DCDPs exhibit, among other things, difficulties with language and social functioning [20], but it is not clear whether these are due to co-occurrence with other developmental disorders, such as SLI and ASD. Young children (but not adults) with DCD exhibit a specific deficit in coherence sensitivity to motion relative to form [115], but it has to be born in mind that these data are from a cross-sectional study; a subset of children with dyslexia and autism also exhibited a deficit on the motion coherence task [116]. Additionally, after controlling for brain size, patients with increasing X or Y chromosome dosage also tend to have a disproportionally reduced size of cerebellum, pallidum and amygdala [117–119]. As discussed above, cerebellar abnormalities have been reported in neuroimaging studies involving DCDAs [51, 52] and children with DCD [82, 120, 121], but also other developmental disorders, such dyslexia [77, 78, 122] and ADHD [123]. Furthermore, studies on children with DCD have revealed functional abnormalities in the basal ganglia and pallidum [124, 125].

A question that has arisen here is why some brain regions get altered when a patient has an additional sex chromosome and others do not. An answer to this question may provide an insight into the disease mechanism. Recent studies suggest a transcriptional vulnerability model, for the spatial targeting of brain, changes in disease. Testing this required mapping anatomical change in neurodevelopmental disorders and then aligning these maps with the Allen Institute Adult Human Microarray Dataset [113]. The results showed that the spatial pattern of anatomical change in each disorder is associated with the spatial expression profile for genes found in the causal CNV region [126]. These results support the view that intrinsic gradients of gene expression in the human brain, shape cortical vulnerability when the gene dosage is altered. A subsequent question here was: what principles of cortical organisation were determining these gene expression gradients? In the search for an answer, the authors [126] collected a comprehensive set of single-cell gene expression signatures and used post-mortem data to map expression gradients for each canonical cell class in the human brain. The results revealed specific cell-classes that expressed CNV genes and closely tracked the spatial pattern of cortical disruption in each disorder, e.g. *MAPK1*-expressing inhibitory neurons in del22q11. This line of research seems very promising and it is likely that it will provide valuable insights into the underlying causes of neurodevelopmental disorders, including DCD.

5. Conclusion

The results from the review of neuroimaging studies on DCDAs presented here, have revealed that this research lags behind that for other developmental disorders. The results suggest that DCDAs' unresolved motor problems from childhood persist into adulthood and are associated with functional and structural brain abnormalities, revealing DCD as a complex developmental disorder with abnormalities across different brain regions. In order to make significant progress in future, it is suggested that further research would need to: (1) focus on a robust theoretical framework; (2) investigate the underlying causes of DCD; (3) use neuroimaging studies based on longitudinal designs; (4) focus on individual differences among DCDAs; (5) extend the types of imaging tools, as well as, if possible, use more than one imaging technique with the same sample of participants with DCD; (6) refine the understanding of environmental factors that increase the risk of DCD and include them in the study design; (7) advance genetics findings on genes, the variants of which increase the risk of developing DCD; (8) focus on neuroimaging intergenerational transmission of brain circuitry; and (9) pursue research on integrative neuroimaging. The current era of incredible technological progress within the field of neuroimaging and molecular genetics must surely result in ground-breaking discoveries in DCD research in the not too distant future.

Acknowledgements

Some of the content reported here was presented at the UK's 7th Biennial Academic and Practitioner Conference on Developmental Coordination Disorder, Brunel University, UK (June 2018). The reviewer's input is gratefully acknowledged.

Conflict of interest

The author declares no conflict of interest.

Author details

Agnieszka Anna Reid
Independent Researcher, Cambridge, UK

*Address all correspondence to: agnieszka.reid@virginmedia.com

References

[1] American Psychiatric Association. Diagnostic and Statistical Manual of Mental Disorders. 5th ed. Arlington, VA: American Psychiatric Association; 2013

[2] Lingam R et al. Prevalence of developmental coordination disorder using the DSM-IV at 7 years of age: A UK population—Based study. Pediatrics. 2009;**123**(4):e693-e700

[3] Kirby A et al. Developmental co-ordination disorder (DCD) in adolescents and adults in further and higher education. Journal of Research in Special Educational Needs. 2008;**8**: 120-131

[4] Sugden DA, Chambers ME. Children with Developmental Coordination Disorder. London: Whurr; 2005

[5] Cousins M, Smyth MM. Developmental coordination impairments in adulthood. Human Movement Science. 2003;**22**(4–5): 433-459

[6] de Oliveira RF, Billington J, Wann JP. Optimal use of visual information in adolescents and young adults with developmental coordination disorder. Experimental Brain Research. 2014; **232**(9):2989-2995

[7] de Oliveira RF, Wann JP. Integration of dynamic information for visuomotor control in young adults with developmental coordination disorder. Experimental Brain Research. 2010; **205**(3):387-394

[8] de Oliveira RF, Wann JP. Driving skills of young adults with developmental coordination disorder: Regulating speed and coping with distraction. Research in Developmental Disabilities. 2011;**32**(4):1301-1308

[9] de Oliveira RF, Wann JP. Driving skills of young adults with developmental coordination disorder: Maintaining control and avoiding hazards. Human Movement Science. 2012;**31**(3):721-729

[10] Du W, Wilmut K, Barnett AL. Level walking in adults with and without developmental coordination disorder: An analysis of movement variability. Human Movement Science. 2015;**43**: 9-14

[11] Gentle J, Barnett AL, Wilmut K. Adaptations to walking on an uneven terrain for individuals with and without developmental coordination disorder. Human Movement Science. 2016;**49**: 346-353

[12] Lee CM, Bo J. Error argumentation enhance adaptability in adults with low motor ability. Journal of Motor Behavior. 2016;**48**(4):297-308

[13] Tal Saban M, Ornoy A, Parush S. Executive function and attention in young adults with and without developmental coordination disorder—A comparative study. Research in Developmental Disabilities. 2014; **35**(11):2644-2650

[14] Wilmut K, Barnett AL. When an object appears unexpectedly: Anticipatory movement and object circumvention in individuals with and without developmental coordination disorder. Experimental Brain Research. 2017;**235**(5):1531-1540

[15] Wilmut K, Byrne M. Grip selection for sequential movements in children and adults with and without developmental coordination disorder. Human Movement Science. 2014;**36**: 272-284

[16] Wilmut K, Byrne M, Barnett AL. Reaching to throw compared to reaching to place: A comparison across individuals with and without

developmental coordination disorder. Research in Developmental Disabilities. 2013;**34**(1):174-182

[17] Wilmut K, Du W, Barnett AL. How do i fit through that gap? Navigation through apertures in adults with and without developmental coordination disorder. PLoS One. 2015;**10**(4): e0124695

[18] Wilmut K, Gentle J, Barnett AL. Gait symmetry in individuals with and without developmental coordination disorder. Research in Developmental Disabilities. 2017;**60**:107-114

[19] Wolpert DM. Probabilistic models of sensorimotor control and decision making. Talairach Lecture given at the 22th Annual Meeting of the OHBM. Geneva, Switzerland. 2016

[20] Dyspraxia Foundation, Dyspraxia: Dyspraxic Adults Surviving in a Non-Dyspraxic World. Kindle ed. Hitchin, UK: Dyspraxia Foundation Adult Support Group; 2015

[21] Kirby A, Edwards L, Sugden DA. Emerging adulthood in developmental co-ordination disorder: Parent and young adult perspectives. Research in Developmental Disabilities. 2011;**32**: 1351-1360

[22] Hill EL, Brown D, Sorgardt KS. A preliminary investigation of quality of life satisfaction reports in emerging adults with and without developmental coordination disorder. Journal of Adult Development. 2011;**18**(3):130-134

[23] Kirby A et al. Self-reported mood, general health, wellbeing and employment status in adults with suspected DCD. Research in Developmental Disabilities. 2013;**34**(4): 1357-1364

[24] Tal-Saban M, Ornoy A, Parush S. Young adults with developmental coordination disorder: A longitudinal study. The American Journal of Occupational Therapy. 2014;**68**(3): 307-316

[25] Thomas M, Christopher G. Fatigue in developmental coordination disorder: An exploratory study in adults. Fatigue: Biomedicine, Health & Behavior. 2017; **6**(1):41-51

[26] Hill EL, Brown D. Mood impairments in adults previously diagnosed with developmental coordination disorder. Journal of Mental Health. 2013;**22**(4):334-340

[27] Waszczuk MA et al. Coordination difficulty and internalizing symptoms in adults: A twin/sibling study. Psychiatry Research. 2016;**239**:1-8

[28] Gagnon-Roy M, Jasmin E, Camden C. Social participation of teenagers and young adults with developmental co-ordination disorder and strategies that could help them: Results from a scoping review. Child: Care, Health and Development. 2016; **42**(6):840-851

[29] Missiuna C et al. Life experiences of young adults who have coordination difficulties. Canadian Journal of Occupational Therapy. 2008;**75**(3): 157-166

[30] Kirby A, Sugden D, Purcell C. Diagnosing developmental coordination disorders. Archives of Disease in Childhood. 2014;**99**(3):292-296

[31] Clark CJ et al. Development and psychometric properties of a screening tool for assessing developmental coordination disorder in adults. International Journal of Physical Medicine & Rehabilitation. 2013;**1**(5):1-9. DOI: 10.4172/2329-9096. 1000145

[32] Kirby A et al. The development and standardization of the adult developmental co-ordination disorders/

dyspraxia checklist (ADC). Research in Developmental Disabilities. 2010;**31**: 131-139

[33] Lichtenstein P et al. The genetics of autism spectrum disorders and related neuropsychiatric disorders in childhood. The American Journal of Psychiatry. 2010;**167**(11):1357-1363

[34] Martin NC, Piek JP, Hay D. DCD and ADHD: A genetic study of their shared aetiology. Human Movement Science. 2006;**25**(1):110-124

[35] Fliers E et al. ADHD and poor motor performance from a family genetic perspective. Journal of the American Academy of Child and Adolescent Psychiatry. 2009;**48**(1):25-34

[36] Fliers EA et al. Genome-wide association study of motor coordination problems in ADHD identifies genes for brain and muscle function. The World Journal of Biological Psychiatry. 2012; **13**(3):211-222

[37] Mosca SJ et al. Copy-number variations are enriched for neurodevelopmental genes in children with developmental coordination disorder. Journal of Medical Genetics. 2016;**53**(12):812-819

[38] Henderson SE, Hall D. Concomitants of clumsiness in young schoolchildren. Developmental Medicine and Child Neurology. 1982; **24**(4):448-460

[39] Piek JP, Rigoli D. In: Cairney J, editor. Psychosocial and Behavioural Difficulties in Children with Developmental Coordination Disorder in Developmental Coordination Disorder and its Consequences. Toronto: University of Toronto Press; 2015

[40] Biotteau M et al. Neural signature of DCD: A critical review of MRI neuroimaging studies. Frontiers in Neurology. 2016;7:227

[41] Peters LH, Maathuis CG, Hadders-Algra M. Neural correlates of developmental coordination disorder. Developmental Medicine and Child Neurology. 2013;**55**(Suppl 4):59-64

[42] Wilson PH et al. Cognitive and neuroimaging findings in developmental coordination disorder: New insights from a systematic review of recent research. Developmental Medicine and Child Neurology. 2017; **59**(11):1117-1129

[43] Zwicker JG et al. Developmental coordination disorder: A review and update. European Journal of Paediatric Neurology. 2012;**16**(6):573-581

[44] Hyde C, Rigoli D, Piek J. Developmental coordination disorder. In: Rinehart N, Bradshaw J, Enticott P, editors. Developmental Disorders of the Brain. London: Psychology Press; 2017

[45] Jones DK, Knosche TR, Turner R. White matter integrity, fiber count, and other fallacies: The do's and don'ts of diffusion MRI. NeuroImage. 2013;**73**: 239-254

[46] Duschek S, Schandry R. Functional transcranial Doppler sonography as a tool in psychophysiological research. Psychophysiology. 2003;**40**(3):436-454

[47] Farquharson S, Tournier JD. High angular resolution diffusion imaging, Diffusion Tensor Imaging. In: Van Hecke W, Emsell L, Sunaert S, editors. A Practical Handbook. New York: Springer; 2016. pp. 383-406

[48] Jones DK, editor. Diffusion MRI. Theory, Methods and Applications. Oxford: Oxford University Press; 2011

[49] Poldrack RA, Mumford JA, Nichols TE. Handbook of Functional MRI Data Analysis. Cambridge: Cambridge University Press; 2011

[50] Toga AW, Mazziotta JC, editors. Brain Mapping: The Methods. 2nd ed. San Diego, USA: Academic Press; 2002

[51] Marien P et al. Developmental coordination disorder: Disruption of the cerebello-cerebral network evidenced by SPECT. Cerebellum. 2010;**9**(3): 405-410

[52] Kashuk SR et al. Diminished motor imagery capability in adults with motor impairment: An fMRI mental rotation study. Behavioural Brain Research. 2017;**334**:86-96

[53] He JL et al. Interhemispheric cortical inhibition is reduced in young adults with developmental coordination disorder. Frontiers in Neurology. 2018; **9**:1-12. DOI: 10.3389/fneur.2018.00179

[54] Hyde C et al. Corticospinal excitability during motor imagery is reduced in young adults with developmental coordination disorder. Research in Developmental Disabilities. 2018;**72**:214-224

[55] Hodgson JC, Hudson JM. Atypical speech lateralization in adults with developmental coordination disorder demonstrated using functional transcranial Doppler ultrasound. Journal of Neuropsychology. 2017;**11**(1):1-13

[56] Williams J et al. White matter alterations in adults with probable developmental coordination disorder: An MRI diffusion tensor imaging study. Neuroreport. 2017;**28**(2):87-92

[57] Hyde C et al. White matter organization in developmental coordination disorder: A pilot study exploring the added value of constrained spherical deconvolution. NeuroImage: Clinical. 2019;**21**:101625

[58] Ashburner J, Friston KJ. Voxel-based morphometry—the methods. NeuroImage. 2000;**11**:805-821

[59] Hyde C et al. Motor imagery is less efficient in adults with probable developmental coordination disorder: Evidence from the hand rotation task. Research in Developmental Disabilities. 2014;**35**(11):3062-3070

[60] Pinel P et al. Genetic variants of FOXP2 and KIAA0319/TTRAP/THEM2 locus are associated with altered brain activation in distinct language-related regions. The Journal of Neuroscience. 2012;**32**(3):817-825

[61] Debrabant J et al. Brain connectomics of visual-motor deficits in children with developmental coordination disorder. The Journal of Pediatrics. 2016;**169**:21-27. e2

[62] Langevin LM et al. Common white matter microstructure alterations in pediatric motor and attention disorders. The Journal of Pediatrics. 2014;**164**(5): 1157-1164 e1

[63] Zwicker JG et al. Developmental coordination disorder: A pilot diffusion tensor imaging study. Pediatric Neurology. 2012;**46**(3):162-167

[64] Jeurissen B et al. Investigating the prevalence of complex fiber configurations in white matter tissue with diffusion magnetic resonance imaging. Human Brain Mapping. 2013; **34**(11):2747-2766

[65] Tournier JD, Mori S, Leemans A. Diffusion tensor imaging and beyond. Magnetic Resonance in Medicine. 2011; **65**(6):1532-1556

[66] Raffelt D et al. Apparent fibre density: A novel measure for the analysis of diffusion-weighted magnetic resonance images. NeuroImage. 2012; **59**(4):3976-3994

[67] Genc S et al. Age, sex, and puberty related development of the corpus callosum: A multi-technique diffusion MRI study. Brain Structure & Function. 2018;**223**(6):2753-2765

[68] Blank R et al. International clinical practice recommendations on the definition, diagnosis, assessment, intervention, and psychosocial aspects of developmental coordination disorder. Developmental Medicine and Child Neurology. 2019;**61**(3):242-285

[69] Evans TM et al. Sex-specific gray matter volume differences in females with developmental dyslexia. Brain Structure & Function. 2014;**219**(3): 1041-1054

[70] Lebel C, Beaulieu C. Longitudinal development of human brain wiring continues from childhood into adulthood. The Journal of Neuroscience. 2011;**31**(30):10937-10947

[71] Taber-Thomas B, Pérez-Edgar K. Emerging adulthood brain development. Arnett JJ, editor. The Oxford Handbook of Emerging Adulthood. Oxford: Oxford University Press; 2016

[72] Kaplan BJ et al. DCD may not be a discrete disorder. Human Movement Science. 1998;**17**:471-490

[73] Dewey D, Bernier FP. The concept of atypical brain development in developmental coordination disorder (DCD)–A new look. Current Developmental Disorders Reports. 2016; **3**(2):161-169

[74] Licari MK, Rigoli D, Piek JP. Biological and genetic factors in DCD. In: Barnett AL, Hill EL, editors. Understanding Motor Behaviour in Developmental Coordination Disorder (Current Issues in Developmental Psychology). Taylor and Francis; 2019. pp. 101-116

[75] Flapper BC, Schoemaker MM. Developmental coordination disorder in children with specific language impairment: Co-morbidity and impact on quality of life. Research in Developmental Disabilities. 2013;**34**(2):756-763

[76] Alloway TP. Working memory, reading, and mathematical skills in children with developmental coordination disorder. Journal of Experimental Child Psychology. 2007; **96**(1):20-36

[77] Reid AA. An fMRI multiple case study of the neural correlates of reading deficit in individuals with developmental dyslexia: Theoretical implications. In: Asher-Hansley V, editor. Advances in Neuroimaging Research. New York: Nova Science Publishers; 2014. pp. 1-119

[78] Reid AA. Neuroimaging reveals heterogeneous neural correlates of reading deficit in individuals with dyslexia consistent with a multiple deficit model. In: Golubic SJ, editor. Neuroimaging: Structure, Function and Mind. Rijeka: IntechOpen; 2019. pp. 1-27. DOI: 10.5772/intechopen.80677

[79] Adams IL et al. Compromised motor control in children with DCD: A deficit in the internal model?—A systematic review. Neuroscience and Biobehavioral Reviews. 2014;**47**:225-244

[80] Wilson PH et al. Toward a hybrid model of developmental coordination disorder. Current Developmental Disorders Reports. 2017;**4**:64-71

[81] Licari MK et al. Cortical functioning in children with developmental coordination disorder: A motor overflow study. Experimental Brain Research. 2015;**233**(6):1703-1710

[82] Zwicker JG et al. Brain activation of children with developmental coordination disorder is different than peers. Pediatrics. 2010;**126**(3): e678-e686

[83] Pennington BF. From single to multiple deficit models of developmental disorders. Cognition. 2006;**101**:385-413

[84] Nicolson RI, Fawcett AJ. Procedural learning difficulties: Reuniting the developmental disorders? Trends in Neurosciences. 2007;**30**(4):135-141

[85] Pugh KR et al. Glutamate and choline levels predict individual differences in reading ability in emergent readers. The Journal of Neuroscience. 2014;**34**(11):4082-4089

[86] Reid AA. A critical review of magnetic resonance spectroscopy (MRS) studies on ADHD. Attention Deficit and Hyperactivity Disorders. 2015;**7**(Suppl 1):34-35

[87] Stagg C, Rothman D. Magnetic Resonance Spectroscopy: Tools for Neuroscience Research and Emerging Clinical Applications. Kindle ed. USA: Elsevier Science; 2014

[88] Gass A, Richards TL. Serial proton magnetic resonance spectroscopy of normal-appearing gray and white matter in MS. Neurology. 2013;**80**(1): 17-18

[89] Geuze RH. Postural control in children with developmental coordination disorder. Neural Plasticity. 2005;**12**(2–3):183-196; discussion 263-72

[90] Boto E et al. A new generation of magnetoencephalography: Room temperature measurements using optically-pumped magnetometers. NeuroImage. 2017;**149**:404-414

[91] Buckner RL, Andrews-Hanna JR, Schacter DL. The Brain's default network: Anatomy, function, and relevance to disease. Annals of the New York Academy of Sciences. 2008; **1124**(1):1-38

[92] Kernbach JM et al. Shared endophenotypes of default mode dsfunction in attention deficit/hyperactivity disorder and autism spectrum disorder. Translational Psychiatry. 2018;**8**(1):133

[93] Kebets V et al. Somatosensory-motor dysconnectivity spans multiple transdiagnostic dimensions of psychopathology. Biological Psychiatry. 2019;**86**:779-791

[94] Hari R, Kujala MV. Brain basis of human social interaction: From concepts to brain imaging. Physiological Reviews. 2009;**89**(2):453-479

[95] Hari R, Parkkonen L. The brain timewise: How timing shapes and supports brain function. Philosophical Transactions of the Royal Society of London. Series B, Biological Sciences. 2015;**370**(1668):1-10. DOI: 10.1098/rstb.2014.0170

[96] Todd N et al. Evaluation of 2D multiband EPI imaging for high-resolution, whole-brain, task-based fMRI studies at 3T: Sensitivity and slice leakage artifacts. Neuroimage. 2016;**124** (Pt A):32-42

[97] De Martino F et al. Frequency preference and attention effects across cortical depths in the human primary auditory cortex. Proceedings of the National Academy of Sciences of the United States of America. 2015;**112**(52): 16036-16041

[98] Faebo Larsen R et al. Determinants of developmental coordination disorder in 7-year-old children: A study of children in the Danish National Birth Cohort. Developmental Medicine and Child Neurology. 2013;**55**(11): 1016-1022

[99] Grace T et al. Early life events and motor development in childhood and adolescence: A longitudinal study. Acta Paediatrica. 2016;**105**(5): e219-e227

[100] Newbury DF. Genetic contributions to neurodevelopmental disorders. In: Barnett AL, Hill EL, editors. Understanding Motor Behaviour in Developmental

Coordination Disorder (Current Issues in Developmental Psychology). Taylor and Francis. 2019. pp. 87-100

[101] Arbogast T et al. Reciprocal effects on neurocognitive and metabolic phenotypes in mouse models of 16p11.2 deletion and duplication syndromes. PLoS Genetics. 2016;**12**(2):e1005709

[102] Ellegood J et al. Neuroanatomical phenotypes in a mouse model of the 22q11.2 microdeletion. Molecular Psychiatry. 2014;**19**(1):99-107

[103] Qian Y, Forssberg H, Diaz Heijtz R. Motor skill learning is associated with phase-dependent modifications in the striatal cAMP/PKA/DARPP-32 signaling pathway in rodents. PLoS One. 2015; **10**(10):e0140974

[104] Gill K et al. Developmental Coordination Disorder: What can we learn from mice? In: 13th International Conference on Developmental Coordination Disorder. Finland: University of Jyväskylä; 2019. p. 53

[105] Parikshak NN, Gandal MJ, Geschwind DH. Systems biology and gene networks in neurodevelopmental and neurodegenerative disorders. Nature Reviews. Genetics. 2015;**16**(8): 441-458

[106] Ho TC et al. Intergenerational neuroimaging of human brain circuitry. Trends in Neurosciences. 2016;**39**(10): 644-648

[107] Yamagata B et al. Female-specific intergenerational transmission patterns of the human corticolimbic circuitry. The Journal of Neuroscience. 2016; **36**(4):1254-1260

[108] Colich NL et al. Like mother like daughter: Putamen activation as a mechanism underlying intergenerational risk for depression. Social Cognitive and Affective Neuroscience. 2017;**12**(9):1480-1489

[109] Raznahan A. Genetics-first approaches in biological psychiatry. Biological Psychiatry. 2018;**84**(4): 234-235

[110] Raznahan A et al. Globally divergent but locally convergent X- and Y-chromosome influences on cortical development. Cerebral Cortex. 2016; **26**(1):70-79

[111] Raznahan A et al. Sex-chromosome dosage effects on gene expression in humans. Proceedings of the National Academy of Sciences of the United States of America. 2018;**115**(28): 7398-7403

[112] Raznahan A. Integrative neuroimaging of the developing brain in health and disease. Paper presented at the 25th Annual Meeting of the Organization for Human Brain Mapping Rome, Itally. 2019

[113] Hawrylycz MJ et al. An anatomically comprehensive atlas of the adult human brain transcriptome. Nature. 2012;**489**(7416):391-399

[114] Amunts K et al. BigBrain: An ultrahigh-resolution 3D human brain model. Science. 2013;**340**(6139): 1472-1475

[115] Corbett FP. Visual Motion Processing in Typical Development and Developmental Coordination Disorder. London: University College; 2017

[116] White S et al. A double dissociation between sensorimotor impairments and reading disability: A comparison of autistic and dyslexic children. Cognitive Neuropsychology. 2006;**23**(5):748-761

[117] Mankiw C et al. Allometric analysis detects Brain size-independent effects of sex and sex chromosome complement on human cerebellar organization. The Journal of Neuroscience. 2017;**37**(21): 5221-5231

[118] Nadig A et al. Carriage of supernumerary sex chromosomes decreases the volume and alters the shape of limbic structures. eNeuro. 2018;**5**(5):1-11. DOI: 10.1523/ENEURO.0265-18.2018

[119] Reardon PK et al. An allometric analysis of sex and sex chromosome dosage effects on subcortical anatomy in humans. The Journal of Neuroscience. 2016;**36**(8):2438-2448

[120] Debrabant J et al. Neural underpinnings of impaired predictive motor timing in children with developmental coordination disorder. Research in Developmental Disabilities. 2013;**34**(5):1478-1487

[121] Zwicker JG et al. Brain activation associated with motor skill practice in children with developmental coordination disorder: An fMRI study. International Journal of Developmental Neuroscience. 2011;**29**(2):145-152

[122] Nicolson RI et al. Association of abnormal cerebellar activation with motor learning difficulties in dyslexic adults. Lancet. 1999;**353**(9165): 1662-1667

[123] Castellanos FX et al. Developmental trajectories of brain volume abnormalities in children and adolescents with attention-deficit/ hyperactivity disorder. JAMA. 2002; **288**(14):1740-1748

[124] McLeod KR et al. Functional connectivity of neural motor networks is disrupted in children with developmental coordination disorder and attention-deficit/hyperactivity disorder. NeuroImage: Clinical. 2014;**4**: 566-575

[125] Querne L et al. Dysfunction of the attentional brain network in children with developmental coordination disorder: A fMRI study. Brain Research. 2008;**1244**:89-102

[126] Seidlitz J et al. Transcriptomic and Cellular Decoding of Regional Brain Vulnerability to Neurodevelopmental Disorders. bioRxiv preprint, 2019. pp. 1-49. DOI: 10.1101/573279

Chapter 4

Electroencephalogram Based Biomarkers for Detection of Alzheimer's Disease

Ali H. Husseen Al-Nuaimi, Shaymaa Al-Juboori, Emmanuel Jammeh, Lingfen Sun and Emmanuel Ifeachor

Abstract

Alzheimer's disease (AD) is an age-related progressive and neurodegenerative disorder, which is characterized by loss of memory and cognitive decline. It is the main cause of disability among older people. The rapid increase in the number of people living with AD and other forms of dementia due to the aging population represents a major challenge to health and social care systems worldwide. Degeneration of brain cells due to AD starts many years before the clinical manifestations become clear. Early diagnosis of AD will contribute to the development of effective treatments that could slow, stop, or prevent significant cognitive decline. Consequently, early diagnosis of AD may also be valuable in detecting patients with dementia who have not obtained a formal early diagnosis, and this may provide them with a chance to access suitable healthcare facilities. An early diagnosis biomarker capable of measuring brain cell degeneration due to AD would be valuable. Potentially, electroencephalogram (EEG) can play a valuable role in the early diagnosis of AD. EEG is noninvasive and low cost, and provides valuable information about brain dynamics in AD. Thus, EEG-based biomarkers may be used as a first-line decision-support tool in AD diagnosis and could complement other AD biomarkers.

Keywords: EEG biomarkers, AD biomarkers, slowing of EEG, decrease in EEG coherence, reduction in EEG complexity, detection of Alzheimer's disease

1. Introduction

Alzheimer's disease (AD) is an age-related progressive neurodegenerative disorder characterized by cognitive impairment and memory loss [1, 2] and is the leading cause of elderly disability [3]. AD is categorized as the sixth major cause of death in the United States among older people [4]. Due to the aging population, the fast growth in the number of individuals living with AD and other kinds of dementia is a major challenge for health and social care systems around the world [5]. There are currently more than 46.8 million people with dementia around the world with an annual care cost estimated at US$ 818 billion and an annual cost of US$ 2 trillion is projected to reach 74.7 million by 2030 [6]. It is estimated that by 2050 the number of people with dementia around the world will exceed 131 million, which will have

 IntechOpen

an enormous financial. However, many dementia sufferers are not diagnosed early [7, 8]. It is estimated that up to 50% of individuals with dementia may not have been diagnosed formally [8, 9]. In 2011, 28 million people out of 36 million people with dementia were not diagnosed worldwide [10].

Degeneration of brain cells due to AD begins many years before clinical manifestations become noticeable [5, 11–15]. Early diagnosis of AD will help to the development of efficient treatments that could mitigate, stop, or prevent significant cognitive impairment [14, 16, 17]. Early diagnosis of AD may also be valuable in detecting patients with dementia who have not obtained a formal early diagnosis, and this may provide them with a chance to access suitable healthcare facilities [18–20].

An early diagnosis biomarker that can measure brain cell degeneration due to AD would be valuable [2, 21–23]. But this may involve dealing with an extremely large number of individuals, as up to 50% of individuals with dementia may not have been diagnosed formally. Therefore, Simple, non-invasive, low-cost and reliable biomarkers are necessary for early diagnosis that can be accessed in clinical practice [5, 24, 25]. Recent guidelines support the use of biomarkers for biochemical and neuroimaging to promote AD diagnosis. AD testing of cerebral spinal fluid (CSF) is not commonly used in clinical practice as it involves lumbar puncture, an invasive procedure [2, 26, 27]. Neuroimaging is expensive, accessible only in specialized centers [28], and may not be appropriate for patients with pacemakers or certain implants [29]. Blood-based biomarkers have shown promising results in the diagnosis of AD but are not yet fully developed and there are currently no low-cost biosensors available for the detection of AD biomarkers in the blood [2, 24, 30].

EEG can play a potential role in early diagnosis of AD [11, 19, 20, 23, 31–33] EEG is non-invasive, low-cost, has a high temporal resolution, and provides valuable information about brain dynamics in AD [19, 20, 32, 34, 35]. The essential utility of EEG in detecting brain signal changes has been proved even at the preclinical stage of the disease [32, 36, 37]. EEG biomarkers can, therefore, be used in the diagnosis of AD as a first-line decision support tool [11, 34] and could supplement other AD biomarkers [25].

As a consequence of brain cell damage that affects brain activity, AD is characterized by memory loss and cognitive impairment [37]. AD leads changes in EEG characteristics [34, 37, 38] and EEG analysis may provide useful information about brain dynamics caused by AD [19, 20, 32, 34]. The most characteristic features in EEG caused by AD are slowing of EEG, a decrease in EEG coherence, and reduction in EEG complexity [32–34, 36–39]. These changes in the EEG can be quantified as a biomarker of AD. In order to quantify EEG changes as AD biomarkers, a range of linear and nonlinear techniques are being developed [40, 41]. AD biomarkers based on EEG slowing and reducing EEG coherence are often produced using linear methods of analysis (i.e. EEG signal spectral analysis) [36, 42, 43]. While biomarkers derived from the EEG complexity analysis are based on non-linear methods (e.g. entropy methods, fractal dimension, and Lempel-Ziv complexity) [44–47].

This chapter describes research into the development of EEG biomarkers that detect AD based on analysis of changes in the EEG. These changes can be quantified as a biomarker of AD. The most characteristic features in EEG caused by AD are slowing of EEG, a decrease in EEG coherence, and reduction in EEG complexity were reviewed in this chapter.

The chapter is arranged as follows. In Section 2, the EEG characteristic features of AD detection. In Section 3, the discussions are presented and the conclusions are presented in Section 4.

2. EEG characteristic features of AD detection

The most characteristic features evident in an EEG that detects AD are slowing of the EEG, a reduction in EEG complexity, and a decrease in EEG coherence [32, 34, 36–39]. These changes can thus be quantified as biomarkers of AD. EEG based biomarkers can therefore be divided into three main categories: the slowing of the EEG, reduction in complexity, and a decrease in the coherence between cortical regions [32–34, 36–39, 48]. The slowing of the EEG and reduction in complexity were reviewed in this chapter.

2.1 Reduction in EEG complexity

Approaches to EEG complexity showed promising results in the diagnosis of AD [11, 34, 49] and seemed suitable for the diagnosis of AD [37, 50, 51]. Complexity is a measure of how random the dynamic behavior of a particular sequence is [52]. The cortical regions of the brain are spontaneously fired, and this dynamic behavior is complex [53, 54]. AD causes a reduction in the neuronal activity of the brain [55] resulting in a decreased ability to process information [56–58] which may be reflected in EEG signals [55]. Several studies have investigated EEG complexity as a potential AD biomarker using whole EEG record with the objective of achieving a high performance. Given the association of EEG activities (e.g., alpha, delta activities) with AD, Al-nuaimi et al. [49] they proved that the derivation of EEG complexity based on EEG activities should lead to enhanced performance. This reduction can be measured using different methods e.g., Tsallis entropy (TsEn) [34, 59, 60], Higuchi Fractal Dimension (HFD) [61], and Lempel Ziv Complexity (LZC) [41, 47]. Consequently, EEG complexity can potentially be a good biomarker for AD diagnosis [37] as AD patients exhibit a significant reduction in EEG complexity [37–39, 48, 55, 62, 63].

In particular, TsEn approach has been shown to be one of the most promising information-theoretic methods for quantifying EEG complexity [34, 59, 60, 64, 65]. It has also been shown to be a reliable analysis tool to use with working memory tasks. Its capacity for rapid computation may serve as the basis for real-time decision support tools for diagnosing AD [34, 59, 65–67]. Sneddon et al. [68] analyzed EEG TsEn and found that it was capable of detecting mild dementia due to AD with 88% for sensitivity and 94% for specificity. De Bock et al. [60] concluded that EEG TsEn was an extremely promising potential diagnostic tool for mild cognitive impairment (MCI) and early dementia with 82% for sensitivity and 73% for specificity. Al-Nuaimi et al. [34] discriminated AD patients with a sensitivity and specificity of 85.8 and 70.9% respectively from normal subjects using the TsEn method. Garn et al. [69] investigated the use of TsEn for the diagnosis of AD on the basis of an EEG analysis and obtained p-value <0.0036 for T7 and T8 channels for discrimination between AD patients and normal subjects.

HFD is a fast computing approach to obtain the fractal dimension of time series signals [70–72] even though there are very few data points available [70]. It can track changes in a biosignal from measuring its complexity [70, 71] and is appropriate for capturing region-specific neural changes due to AD [43, 72]. Furthermore, HFD offers a precise measure of the complexity of the signal compared to other methods [44, 70, 73] and has been shown to be an effective approach to discriminate between AD patients and normal subjects [30, 61]. HFD of the EEG is potentially a useful biomarker of AD diagnosis as it is significantly smaller in AD patients than in normal subjects [49, 61, 74]. Smits et al. [61] discovered that HFD is sensitive to neural changes selectively related in patients with AD and normal subjects. Al-nuaimi et al. [49] analyzed HFD of EEG for AD detection and discovered that HFD is a promising EEG biomarker that captures changes in brain areas thought to be first affected by AD and could be used to identify AD with sensitivity and specificity values of 100 and 80% respectively.

LZC is a nonparametric and nonlinear method that provides a powerful method for quantifying the complexity of finite length sequences [75, 76]. It has previously been used to analyze EEG complexity in patients with AD [41, 77]. The reduction of LZC values may therefore be a good biomarker for AD [41, 77, 78]. It is a simple and powerful approach used in a number of biomedical applications [76]. LZC relies on coarse-grain measurement processing [77], and can be directly applied to the physiological signal without pre-processing [78]. LZC has been extensively used to measure the complexity of discrete-time physiological signals in the analysis of biomedical signals (e.g. EEG) [75]. It is also used in patients with AD to analyze brain function, transmission of brain information, and EEG complexity in patients with AD [41]. The LZC method produces a good biomarker for AD detection [78, 79]. Using LZC in AD patients, Hornero et al. [80] analyzed EEG and magnetoencephalogram (MEG). They discovered that LZC provides a useful insight into the EEG background activity features and the changes related to AD. Hornero et al. [81] discovered that LZC values were smaller in AD patients and proposed that the most significant differences were in the posterior region. In addition, they proposed that a reduced degree of irregularity and complexity characterize the MEG activity of AD patients and that LZC measurements can be used to identify AD patients with a sensitivity and specificity of 65 and 76.2% respectively. McBride et al. [62] investigated the complexity of EEG based on LZC approach for discriminating between patients with early cognitive impairment (MCI), AD patients and normal subjects. They discovered EEG complexity characteristics to provide promising results in discriminating between MCI, AD, and normal subjects for particular EEG frequency bands with regional electrical activity. The complexity of MEG in MCI patients, AD patients and normal subjects was investigated by Fernandez et al. [82] based on the LZC approach of discriminating between the three groups. They discovered that they could differentiate between AD patients and MCI patients with 94.4% for sensitivity and specificity by combining age and posterior LZC scores.

2.2 Slowing of EEG

The slowing of the EEG is one of the most consistent features relating to the detection of AD. Slowing may therefore be quantified as a biomarker of AD [11, 37, 83]. It can be measured in several ways such as changes in EEG amplitude (ΔEEG_A), zero-crossing intervals (ZCI) [11], and changes in the power spectrum (ΔPS) of the EEG signal [11, 32, 33, 37, 39, 84–91]. Al-nuaimi et al. [5] quantified slowing in EEG by measuring the ΔEEG_A. Their results showed that ΔEEG_A is a promising nonlinear EEG marker in the time domain. It can be measured through changes in EEG amplitude and can track changes in the EEG over time [5]. Their results showed that a gradual change in EEG amplitude is a marker for the subsequent rate of cognitive and functional decline in AD patients [5]. The reduction of ZCI of an EEG signal has also been shown to be a promising biomarker of AD [11, 74]. The slowing of the EEG can also be quantified by the power of the EEG signal in different frequency bands (i.e., delta, theta, alpha, beta, and gamma) where slowing is manifest in a decrease in power of high-frequency bands (alpha and beta) and an increase in power of low-frequency bands (delta and theta). These changes can be used to distinguish AD patients from those with other types of dementia [11, 32, 33, 37, 39].

An increase in the power ratio of the alpha/middle alpha bands is an indicator of mild cognitive impairment (MCI) in people who may go on to develop AD [87]. Conversely, an increase in the power ratio of theta/gamma bands has been associated with MCI patients who may not develop AD [92]. This increase was related to a decline in memory and can therefore be used to identify MCI patients in a cohort of normal people [36]. Numerous studies have shown that power changes in the EEG frequency bands are promising markers of AD [84–91].

2.3 Reduction in EEG coherence

AD causes changes in the cortical activity of the brain [93] which impacts the connectivity among cortical regions of the brain [37], which can be reflected in the EEG coherence. EEG coherence can be quantified by assessing the functional coupling between brain regions [37, 94]. Coherence measures depend on channel location and the frequency bands of the EEG signal [93, 95–98]. Studies have shown that AD patients have a significant reduction in the coherence in the alpha band especially in the temporo-parieto-occipital regions and an increase in the coherence in the delta band [93]. Furthermore, AD patients have a significant increase in the high beta band and a decrease in the delta band [99]. AD patients have also a reduction in both the left temporal alpha band and interhemispheric theta band compared to normal [97]. In addition, a positive association has been shown in EEG coherence in the frontal region for delta and beta bands [96]. The EEG coherence has been shown to be a sensitive and selective method for assessing the integrity of structural connections between brain areas in AD patients [98].

3. Discussions

Damage to nerve cells/pathways in the brain due to AD causes changes in the information-processing activity of the brain. These changes are thought to be reflected in the information content of the EEG. Therefore, each analysis technique of EEG signal may capture a different characteristic e.g., complexity, slowing, and coherence of the EEG signal. However, for each technique, there are different analysis methods and each method may measure a different feature that related to cognitive decline in the brain due to AD. Therefore, each method has a different performance. High-performance result referring the used techniques and biomarkers were accurate enough, this provides an indicator for using them in the future studies, and may also be possible to test the candidate biomarkers and techniques in regular health checkup performed by clinicians.

Unlike previous researches, Al-Nuaimi et al. [48], concluded that the complexity measures extracted from the EEG frequency bands (i.e. delta, theta, alpha, beta, and gamma) provide significantly better efficiency in the detection of AD than those extracted from the entire EEG record. This is due to the significant differences between the complexity measurements for AD patients and normal subjects when extracted from the frequency bands compared to the entire record, which is the desirable property of a good biomarker. In particular, they discovered that the best performance was provided by the complexity measurements extracted from the delta and gamma bands for TsEn and HFD. Three EEG channels (T4, O1, and O2) have provided the best performance for the delta band. While F4 has provided the best performance for the theta band.

Similar results for the LZC's complexity measures were achieved, except that C3 was the best EEG channel for the theta band. This is consistent with the results of other researches proposing that AD starts at the back of the brain and then gradually extends to other areas of the brain [5, 49, 83, 100, 101]. This means that AD can be detected using only a small number of EEG channels.

Their results suggest that the three EEG complexity measures, derived from the EEG frequency bands, can detect AD reliably (with sensitivity and specificity of >90%). Thus, EEG complexity measures could provide a basis for developing an accurate, low-cost and easy use tool to detect AD.

They found that AD patients have significantly lower complexity measures for specific EEG frequency bands and for specific EEG channels than normal subjects. This is consistent with findings of in previous studies [32–34, 36–39]. Thus, specific EEG channels and specific frequency bands can be identified which can provide the best biomarkers for the detection of AD. This can be used to achieve good performance in situations where the number of channels available is limited (e.g. when portable EEG systems are used outside specialist centers).

Al-nuaimi et al. [5] developed a new approach for detecting AD based on analyzing changes in EEG amplitude (ΔEEG_A). Their results suggested that ΔEEG_A is a promising biomarker for AD. As AD subjects have significantly lower ΔEEG_A values., this provides an effective way to discriminate between AD patients and normal subjects. The reduction in ΔEEG_A values is thought to be due to the slowing in the EEG as a result of AD and this is in keeping with the finding in other studies [102].

The findings of their studies have a number of implications for research to develop new and robust techniques for the analysis of EEG to increase the contributions EEG makes to the diagnosis of AD.

Several biomarkers were developed for AD diagnosis. However, some of these studies investigated the rationality of combining multiple biomarkers in one diagnostic index [2, 103–105]. Poil et al. [104] investigated the performance of six EEG based biomarkers separately and they combined them in one diagnostic model. They found, combining multiple biomarkers could be more sensitive for early diagnosis of AD. Polikar et al. [106] combined EEG, MRI and PET biomarkers. They suggested the combination of different biomarkers could improve the diagnostic accuracy over any of the individual data sources. Walhovd et al. [107] found combining MR and CSF biomarkers can improve diagnostic classification of AD. Consequently, combining multiple biomarkers from different analysis methods in one diagnostic index may assist to increase the diagnostic performance.

AD is the most common form of dementia and many dementia sufferers do not receive an early diagnosis. Currently, no specific device is available to diagnose AD. Therefore, developing new biomarkers or combining multiple biomarkers to produce a new biomarker with high performance may contribute to the development of robust diagnosis methods that can be used to develop a new specific application for AD diagnosis in its early stages. Furthermore, early diagnosis of AD will contribute to the development of effective treatments that could slow, stop or prevent significant cognitive decline.

4. Conclusions

AD causes changes in the EEG due to memory loss and cognitive impairment, and these changes are thought to be associated with functional disconnections between cortical regions caused by brain cell death [37]. EEG assessment can, therefore, provide useful information on brain dynamics in AD. AD causes a decrease in brain neuronal activity that can be reflected in EEG signals. Non-linear approaches based on EEG complexity methods showed promising results in the detected EEG changes that were thought to be due to AD [5, 34, 48, 49].

EEG based biomarkers can be used as the first line of decision making because these biomarkers are non-invasive, and low cost compared to others e.g., CSF, MRI or PET. However, EEG based biomarkers can complement other biomarkers [25, 106, 108].

EEG based biomarkers to detect AD have some limitations such as the size of samples were used in each study. Most of the EEG studies used a data sized between 10 and 100 of samples [109], unlike the MRI biomarkers, have thousands of samples available with free access as shown in ADNI dataset [4]. Most of the used EEG samples are cross-section, not a longitudinal dataset, and not free access to EEG datasets of AD. To overcome those limitations, longitudinal EEG dataset of AD may assist to track the dynamic changes in the brain which caused by AD, a large number of EEG sample may help to add more reality to the results, and free access to EEG dataset of AD will minimize the burden that researchers spent in collecting the dataset.

In this study, we reviewed an important class of complexity measures, information-theoretic methods, which offers a potentially powerful approach for quantifying changes in the EEG due to AD [59]. Information-theoretic methods have emerged as a potentially useful complexity-based approach to derive robust EEG biomarkers of AD [50, 59, 60, 65, 110, 111]. They are attractive due to the potential natural connection between biomarkers based on information theory and brain changes induced by AD [59]. Conceptually, information-processing activities in the brain are considered to be reflected in the information content of the EEG.

As a result, EEG complexity can potentially be a useful biomarker for the diagnosis of AD. We examined the three complexity measures approached by TsEn, HFD, and LZC extracted from the EEG frequency bands. TsEn, HFD, and LZC values in AD patients were found to be significantly lower in AD patients than in normal subjects for specific EEG frequency bands and specific EEG channels.

This study demonstrates that the complexity measures can detect the abnormalities induced by AD. However, other neurodegenerative diseases, such as other kinds of dementia, may cause similar changes. To improve the diagnostic usefulness of the methods, further development may be necessary to distinguish between dementias.

The slowing of the EEG was also reviewed. It is one of the most consistent features relating to the detection of AD. The slowing of EEG may therefore be quantified as a biomarker of AD [11, 37, 83].

Conflict of interest

The authors declare that there are no conflicts of interest regarding the publication of this article.

Author details

Ali H. Husseen Al-Nuaimi[1*], Shaymaa Al-Juboori[2], Emmanuel Jammeh[2], Lingfen Sun[2] and Emmanuel Ifeachor[2]

1 College of Education for Pure Science (Ibn Al-Haitham), University of Baghdad, Baghdad, Iraq

2 School of Engineering, Computing and Mathematics, Faculty of Science and Engineering, University of Plymouth, Plymouth, United Kingdom

*Address all correspondence to: ali.al-nuaimi@plymouth.ac.uk

References

[1] Harmony T, Fernández T, Gersenowies J, Galán L, Fernández-Bouzas A, Aubert E, et al. Specific EEG frequencies signal general common cognitive processes as well as specific task processes in man. International Journal of Psychophysiology. 2004;**53**(3):207-216

[2] Humpel C. Identifying and validating biomarkers for Alzheimer's disease. Trends in Biotechnology. 2011;**29**(1):26-32

[3] World Health Organization. WHO Mental Health Gap Action Programme (mhGAP) 2008. 2014

[4] ADNI, Alzheimer's Disease Neuroimaging Initiative [Internet]. Available from: http://www.adni-info.org/Home.html

[5] Al-nuaimi AH, Jammeh E, Sun L, Ifeachor E. Changes in the EEG amplitude as a biomarker for early detection of Alzheimer's disease. In: Engineering in Medicine and Biology Society (EMBC), 2016 IEEE 38th Annual International Conference of the IEEE. 2016. pp. 993-996

[6] Prince M, Anders W, Maëlenn G, Ali G-C, Yu-Tzu W, Matthew P. World Alzheimer Report [Internet]. 2015. Available from: https://www.alz.co.uk/research/WorldAlzheimerReport2015.pdf

[7] Prince M, Comas-Herrera A, Knapp M, Guerchet M, Karagiannidou M. World Alzheimer Report 2016 Improving Healthcare for People Living with Dementia. Coverage, Quality and Costs Now and in the Future. 2016. pp. 1-140. Available from: https://www.alz.co.uk/research/world-report-2016

[8] Jammeh E, Carroll C, Pearson S, Escudero J, Anastasiou A, Zajicek J, et al. Using NHS primary care data to identify undiagnosed dementia. Journal of Neurology, Neurosurgery, and Psychiatry. 2015;**86**(11):e4-e4

[9] Michalowsky B, Eichler T, Thyrian JR, Hertel J, Wucherer D, Hoffmann W, et al. Healthcare resource utilization and cost in dementia: Are there differences between patients screened positive for dementia with and those without a formal diagnosis of dementia in primary care in Germany? International Psychogeriatrics. 2016;**28**(03):359-369

[10] Prince M, Bryce R, Ferri C. World Alzheimer Report 2011: The Benefits of Early Diagnosis and Intervention. Alzheimer's Disease International; 2011

[11] Henderson G, Ifeachor E, Hudson N, Goh C, Outram N, Wimalaratna S, et al. Development and assessment of methods for detecting dementia using the human electroencephalogram. IEEE Transactions on Biomedical Engineering. 2006;**53**(8):1557-1568

[12] AL S, editor. Alzheimer Disease Sourcebook. 5th ed. Detroit, Omnigraphics: Peter E. Ruffner; 2011

[13] Galimberti D, Scarpani E, editors. Biomarkers for Early Diagnosis of Alzheimer's Disease. Galimberti: Nova Biomedical Books; 2008

[14] Association A. 2016 Alzheimer's disease facts and figures. Alzheimer's & Dementia. 2017;**12**(4):459-509

[15] Jellinger KA, Janetzky B, Attems J, Kienzl E. Biomarkers for early diagnosis of Alzheimer disease: 'Alzheimer Associated gene'–a new blood biomarker? Journal of Cellular and Molecular Medicine. 2008;**12**(4):1094-1117

[16] Ritchie K, Lovestone S. The dementias. The Lancet. 2002;**360**(9347):1759-1766

[17] Sperling RA, Aisen PS, Beckett LA, Bennett DA, Craft S, Fagan AM, et al. Toward defining the preclinical stages of Alzheimer's disease: Recommendations from the National Institute on Aging-Alzheimer's association workgroups on diagnostic guidelines for Alzheimer's disease. Alzheimer's & Dementia. 2011;7(3):280-292

[18] Greicius MD, Krasnow B, Reiss AL, Menon V. Functional connectivity in the resting brain: A network analysis of the default mode hypothesis. Proceedings of the National Academy of Sciences. 2003;**100**(1):253-258

[19] Gevins A, Smith ME, McEvoy L, Yu D. High-resolution EEG mapping of cortical activation related to working memory: Effects of task difficulty, type of processing, and practice. Cerebral Cortex. 1997;**7**(4):374-385

[20] Sasaki K, Nambu A, Tsujimoto T, Matsuzaki R, Kyuhou S, Gemba H. Studies on integrative functions of the human frontal association cortex with MEG. Cognitive Brain Research. 1996;**5**(1):165-174

[21] Abeel T, Helleputte T, Van de Peer Y, Dupont P, Saeys Y. Robust biomarker identification for cancer diagnosis with ensemble feature selection methods. Bioinformatics. 2010;**26**(3):392-398

[22] Boucheham A, Batouche M. Robust biomarker discovery for cancer diagnosis based on meta-ensemble feature selection. In: Science and Information Conference (SAI), 2014. IEEE. 2014. pp. 452-560

[23] Al-nuaimi AH, Jammeh E, Sun L, Ifeachor E. Changes in the electroencephalogram as a biomarker of Alzheimer 's disease. In: Biosense Dementia 2017 – International Workshop on Biosensors for Dementia from 13 – 14 June 2017 – Plymouth University. Plymouth, UK: International Workshop on Biosensors for Dementia; 2017. p. 40. Available from: https://www.plymouth.ac.uk/whats-on/biosense-dementia

[24] Cedazo-Minguez A, Winblad B. Biomarkers for Alzheimer's disease and other forms of dementia: Clinical needs, limitations and future aspects. Experimental Gerontology. 2010;**45**(1):5-14

[25] Ferreira D, Jelic V, Cavallin L, Oeksengaard A-R, Snaedal J, Høgh P, et al. Electroencephalography is a good complement to currently established dementia biomarkers. Dementia and Geriatric Cognitive Disorders. 2016;**42**(1-2):80-92

[26] Blennow K, Hampel H. CSF markers for incipient Alzheimer's disease. Lancet Neurology. 2003;**2**(10):605-613

[27] O'Bryant SE, Mielke MM, Rissman RA, Lista S, Vanderstichele H, Zetterberg H, et al. Blood-based biomarkers in Alzheimer disease: Current state of the science and a novel collaborative paradigm for advancing from discovery to clinic. Alzheimer's & Dementia. 2017;**13**(1):45-58

[28] Ferreira D, Perestelo-Pérez L, Westman E, Wahlund L-O, Sarría A, Serrano-Aguilar P. Meta-review of CSF core biomarkers in Alzheimer's disease: The state-of-the-art after the new revised diagnostic criteria. Frontiers in Aging Neuroscience. 2014;**6**:47

[29] Weiner M, Khachaturian Z. The Use of MRI and PET for Clinical Diagnosis of Dementia and Investigation of Cognitive Impairment: A Consensus Report. Alzheimer's Assoc Chicago; 2005

[30] Dubois B, Hampel H, Feldman HH, Scheltens P, Aisen P, Andrieu S, et al. Preclinical Alzheimer's disease: Definition, natural history, and diagnostic criteria. Alzheimer's & Dementia. 2016;**12**(3):292-323

[31] Jiang H, White MP, Greicius MD, Waelde LC, Spiegel D. Brain activity and functional connectivity associated with hypnosis. Cerebral Cortex. 2016;**27**(8):4083-4093

[32] Signorino M, Pucci E, Belardinelli N, Nolfe G, Angeleri F. EEG spectral analysis in vascular and Alzheimer dementia. Electroencephalography and Clinical Neurophysiology. 1995;**94**(5):313-325

[33] Besthorn C, Zerfass R, Geiger-Kabisch C, Sattel H, Daniel S, Schreiter-Gasser U, et al. Discrimination of Alzheimer's disease and normal aging by EEG data. Electroencephalography and Clinical Neurophysiology. 1997;**103**(2):241-248

[34] Al-Nuaimi AH, Jammeh E, Sun L, Ifeachor E. Tsallis entropy as a biomarker for detection of Alzheimer's disease. In: Engineering in Medicine and Biology Society (EMBC), 2015 37th Annual International Conference of the IEEE. IEEE; 2015. pp. 4166-4169

[35] Horvath A, Szucs A, Csukly G, Sakovics A, Stefanics G, Kamondi A. EEG and ERP biomarkers of Alzheimer's disease: a critical review. Frontiers in Bioscience. 2018;**23**:183-220

[36] Moretti DV, Fracassi C, Pievani M, Geroldi C, Binetti G, Zanetti O, et al. Increase of theta/gamma ratio is associated with memory impairment. Clinical Neurophysiology. 2009;**120**(2):295-303

[37] Jeong J. EEG dynamics in patients with Alzheimer's disease. Clinical Neurophysiology. 2004;**115**(7):1490-1505

[38] Latchoumane C-FV, Ifeachor E, Hudson N, Wimalaratna S, Jeong J. Dynamical nonstationarity analysis of resting EEGs in Alzheimer's disease. In: International Conference on Neural Information Processing. Springer; 2007. pp. 921-929

[39] Dauwels J, Vialatte F-B, Cichocki A. On the early diagnosis of Alzheimer's disease from EEG signals: A mini-review. In: Advances in Cognitive Neurodynamics (II). Dordrecht: Springer; 2011. pp. 709-716

[40] Babiloni C, Binetti G, Cassetta E, Dal Forno G, Del Percio C, Ferreri F, et al. Sources of cortical rhythms change as a function of cognitive impairment in pathological aging: A multicenter study. Clinical Neurophysiology. 2006;**117**(2):252-268

[41] Abásolo D, Hornero R, Gómez C, García M, López M. Analysis of EEG background activity in Alzheimer's disease patients with Lempel–Ziv complexity and central tendency measure. Medical Engineering & Physics. 2006;**28**(4):315-322

[42] Babiloni C, Del Percio C, Vecchio F, Sebastiano F, Di Gennaro G, Quarato PP, et al. Alpha, beta and gamma electrocorticographic rhythms in somatosensory, motor, premotor and prefrontal cortical areas differ in movement execution and observation in humans. Clinical Neurophysiology. 2016;**127**(1):641-654

[43] Yener GG, Emek-Savaş DD, Lizio R, Çavuşoğlu B, Carducci F, Ada E, et al. Frontal delta event-related oscillations relate to frontal volume in mild cognitive impairment and healthy controls. International Journal of Psychophysiology. 2016;**103**:110-117

[44] Gómez C, Mediavilla Á, Hornero R, Abásolo D, Fernández A. Use of the Higuchi's fractal dimension for the analysis of MEG recordings from Alzheimer's disease patients. Medical Engineering & Physics. 2009;**31**(3):306-313

[45] Labate D, La Foresta F, Morabito G, Palamara I, Morabito FC. Entropic measures of EEG complexity in Alzheimer's disease through a

multivariate multiscale approach. IEEE Sensors Journal. 2013;**13**(9):3284-3292

[46] Lin P-F, Lo M-T, Tsao J, Chang Y-C, Lin C, Ho Y-L. Correlations between the signal complexity of cerebral and cardiac electrical activity: A multiscale entropy analysis. PLoS One. 2014;**9**(2):e87798

[47] Simons S, Abasolo D, Hughes M. Investigation of Alzheimer's disease EEG frequency components with Lempel-Ziv complexity. In: 6th European Conference of the International Federation for Medical and Biological Engineering. Springer; 2015. pp. 46-49

[48] Al-Nuaimi AHH, Jammeh E, Sun L, Ifeachor E. Complexity measures for quantifying changes in electroencephalogram in Alzheimer's disease. Complexity. 2018;**2018**:1-12. Available from: https://www.hindawi.com/journals/complexity/2018/8915079/

[49] Al-nuaimi AH, Jammeh E, Sun L, Ifeachor E. Higuchi fractal dimension of the electroencephalogram as a biomarker for early detection of Alzheimer's disease. In: Engineering in Medicine and Biology Society (EMBC), 2017 IEEE 39th Annual International Conference of the IEEE. IEEE; 2017. pp. 2320-2324

[50] Abásolo D, Hornero R, Espino P, Poza J, Sánchez CI, de la Rosa R. Analysis of regularity in the EEG background activity of Alzheimer's disease patients with approximate entropy. Clinical Neurophysiology. 2005;**116**(8):1826-1834

[51] Kantz H, Schreiber T. Nonlinear Time Series Analysis. 2nd ed. Cambridge, UK: Cambridge University Press; 2004

[52] Lempel A, Ziv J. On the complexity of finite sequences. IEEE Transactions on Information Theory. 1976;**22**(1):75-81

[53] Tononi G, Edelman GM, Sporns O. Complexity and coherency: Integrating information in the brain. Trends in Cognitive Sciences. 1998;**2**(12):474-484

[54] Wackerbauer R, Witt A, Atmanspacher H, Kurths J, Scheingraber H. A comparative classification of complexity measures. Chaos, Solitons & Fractals. 1994;**4**(1):133-173

[55] Besthorn C, Sattel H, Geiger-Kabisch C, Zerfass R, Förstl H. Parameters of EEG dimensional complexity in Alzheimer's disease. Electroencephalography and Clinical Neurophysiology. 1995;**95**(2):84-89

[56] Burgess AP, Rehman J, Williams JD. Changes in neural complexity during the perception of 3D images using random dot stereograms. International Journal of Psychophysiology. 2003;**48**(1):35-42

[57] Gu F, Meng X, Shen E, Cai Z. Can we measure consciousness with EEG complexities? International Journal of Bifurcation and Chaos. 2003;**13**(03):733-742

[58] Adeli H, Ghosh-Dastidar S. Automated EEG-Based Diagnosis of Neurological Disorders: Inventing the Future of Neurology. Boca Raton: CRC Press; 2010

[59] Zhao P, Van-Eetvelt P, Goh C, Hudson N, Wimalaratna S, Ifeachor E. Characterization of EEGs in Alzheimer's disease using information theoretic methods. In: Engineering in Medicine and Biology Society, 2007 EMBS 2007 29th Annual International Conference of the IEEE. IEEE; 2007. pp. 5127-5131

[60] De Bock TJ, Das S, Mohsin M, Munro NB, Hively LM, Jiang Y, et al.

Early detection of Alzheimer's disease using nonlinear analysis of EEG via Tsallis entropy. In: Biomedical Sciences and Engineering Conference (BSEC), 2010. IEEE; 2010. pp. 1-4

[61] Smits FM, Porcaro C, Cottone C, Cancelli A, Rossini PM, Tecchio F. Electroencephalographic fractal dimension in healthy ageing and Alzheimer's disease. PLoS One. 2016;**11**(2):e0149587

[62] McBride JC, Zhao X, Munro NB, Smith CD, Jicha GA, Hively L, et al. Spectral and complexity analysis of scalp EEG characteristics for mild cognitive impairment and early Alzheimer's disease. Computer Methods and Programs in Biomedicine. 2014;**114**(2):153-163

[63] Dauwels J, Srinivasan K, Ramasubba Reddy M, Musha T, Vialatte F-B, Latchoumane C, et al. Slowing and loss of complexity in Alzheimer's EEG: Two sides of the same coin? International Journal of Alzheimer's Disease. 2011;**2011**:539621

[64] Dauwels J, Vialatte F, Cichocki A. Diagnosis of Alzheimer's disease from EEG signals: Where are we standing? Current Alzheimer Research. 2010;7(6):487-505

[65] Hamadicharef B, Guan C, Ifeachor E, Hudson N, Wimalaratna S. Performance evaluation and fusion of methods for early detection of Alzheimer disease. In: BioMedical Engineering and Informatics, 2008 BMEI 2008 International Conference on IEEE. 2008. pp. 347-351

[66] Al-Qazzaz NK, Ali S, Ahmad SA, Islam MS, Escudero J. Entropy-based markers of EEG background activity of stroke-related mild cognitive impairment and vascular dementia patients. In Sensors and electronic instrumentation advances: proceedings of the 2nd international conference on sensors and electronic instrumentation advances 2016. pp. 22-23

[67] Coronel C, Garn H, Waser M, Deistler M, Benke T, Dal-Bianco P, et al. Quantitative EEG markers of entropy and auto mutual information in relation to MMSE scores of probable Alzheimer's disease patients. Entropy. 2017;**19**(3):130

[68] Sneddon R, Shankle WR, Hara J, Rodriquez A, Hoffman D, Saha U. EEG detection of early Alzheimer's disease using psychophysical tasks. Clinical EEG and Neuroscience. 2005;**36**(3):141-150

[69] Garn H, Waser M, Deistler M, Benke T, Dal-Bianco P, Ransmayr G, et al. Quantitative EEG markers relate to Alzheimer's disease severity in the prospective dementia registry Austria (PRODEM). Clinical Neurophysiology. 2015;**126**(3):505-513

[70] Accardo A, Affinito M, Carrozzi M, Bouquet F. Use of the fractal dimension for the analysis of electroencephalographic time series. Biological Cybernetics. 1997;77(5):339-350

[71] Preißl H, Lutzenberger W, Pulvermüller F, Birbaumer N. Fractal dimensions of short EEG time series in humans. Neuroscience Letters. 1997;**225**(2):77-80

[72] Higuchi T. Approach to an irregular time series on the basis of the fractal theory. Physica D: Nonlinear Phenomena. 1988;**31**(2):277-283

[73] Esteller R, Vachtsevanos G, Echauz J. Lilt B. A comparison of fractal dimension algorithms using synthetic and experimental data. In: Circuits and Systems, 1999 ISCAS'99 Proceedings of the 1999 IEEE International Symposium on IEEE. 1999. pp. 199-202

[74] Staudinger T, Polikar R. Analysis of complexity based EEG features for the diagnosis of Alzheimer's disease. In: Engineering in Medicine and Biology Society, EMBC, 2011 Annual International Conference of the IEEE. IEEE; 2011. pp. 2033-2036

[75] Abásolo D, Simons S, da Silva RM, Tononi G, Vyazovskiy VV. Lempel-Ziv complexity of cortical activity during sleep and waking in rats. Journal of Neurophysiology. 2015;**113**(7):2742-2752

[76] Rivolta MW, Migliorini M, Aktaruzzaman M, Sassi R, Bianchi AM. Effects of the series length on Lempel-Ziv complexity during sleep. In: Engineering in Medicine and Biology Society (EMBC), 2014 36th Annual International Conference of the IEEE. IEEE; 2014. pp. 693-696

[77] Zhang X-S, Roy RJ, Jensen EW. EEG complexity as a measure of depth of anesthesia for patients. IEEE Transactions on Biomedical Engineering. 2001;**48**(12):1424-1433

[78] Aboy M, Hornero R, Abásolo D, Álvarez D. Interpretation of the Lempel-Ziv complexity measure in the context of biomedical signal analysis. IEEE Transactions on Biomedical Engineering. 2006;**53**(11):2282-2288

[79] Simons S, Abásolo D. Distance-based Lempel–Ziv complexity for the analysis of electroencephalograms in patients with Alzheimer's disease. Entropy. 2017;**19**(3):129

[80] Hornero R, Abásolo D, Escudero J, Gómez C. Nonlinear analysis of electroencephalogram and magnetoencephalogram recordings in patients with Alzheimer's disease. Philosophical Transactions of the Royal Society A: Mathematical, Physical and Engineering Sciences. 2009;**367**(1887):317-336

[81] Hornero R, Escudero J, Fernández A, Poza J, Gómez C. Spectral and nonlinear analyses of MEG background activity in patients with Alzheimer's disease. IEEE Transactions on Biomedical Engineering. 2008;**55**(6):1658-1665

[82] Fernandez A, Hornero R, Gomez C, Turrero A, Gil-Gregorio P, Matías-Santos J, et al. Complexity analysis of spontaneous brain activity in Alzheimer disease and mild cognitive impairment: An MEG study. Alzheimer Disease and Associated Disorders. 2010;**24**(2):182-189

[83] Babiloni C, Ferri R, Binetti G, Vecchio F, Frisoni GB, Lanuzza B, et al. Directionality of EEG synchronization in Alzheimer's disease subjects. Neurobiology of Aging. 2009;**30**(1):93-102

[84] Babiloni C, Del Percio C, Capotosto P, Noce G, Infarinato F, Muratori C, et al. Cortical sources of resting state electroencephalographic rhythms differ in relapsing–remitting and secondary progressive multiple sclerosis. Clinical Neurophysiology. 2016;**127**(1):581-590

[85] Moretti DV. Electro encephalography-driven approach to prodromal Alzheimer's disease diagnosis: From biomarker integration to network-level comprehension. Clinical Interventions in Aging. 2016;**11**:897

[86] Klimesch W. EEG alpha and theta oscillations reflect cognitive and memory performance: A review and analysis. Brain Research Reviews. 1999;**29**(2):169-195

[87] Moretti DV. Association of EEG, MRI, and regional blood flow biomarkers is predictive of prodromal Alzheimer's disease. Neuropsychiatric Disease and Treatment. 2015;**11**:2779

[88] Moretti DV, Frisoni GB, Binetti G, Zanetti O. Comparison of the effects of transdermal and oral rivastigmine on cognitive function and EEG markers in patients with Alzheimer's disease. Frontiers in Aging Neuroscience. 2014;**6**:179

[89] Kanda PAM, Oliveira EF. Fraga FJ. EEG epochs with less alpha rhythm improve discrimination of mild Alzheimer's. Computer Methods and Programs in Biomedicine. 2017;**138**:13-22

[90] Babiloni C, Lizio R, Del Percio C, Marzano N, Soricelli A, Salvatore E, et al. Cortical sources of resting state EEG rhythms are sensitive to the progression of early stage Alzheimer's disease. Journal of Alzheimer's Disease. 2013;**34**(4):1015-1035

[91] Babiloni C, Lizio R, Marzano N, Capotosto P, Soricelli A, Triggiani AI, et al. Brain neural synchronization and functional coupling in Alzheimer's disease as revealed by resting state EEG rhythms. International Journal of Psychophysiology. 2016;**103**:88-102

[92] Moretti DV, Paternicò D, Binetti G, Zanetti O, Frisoni GB. EEG markers are associated to gray matter changes in thalamus and basal ganglia in subjects with mild cognitive impairment. NeuroImage. 2012;**60**(1):489-496

[93] Locatelli T, Cursi M, Liberati D, Franceschi M, Comi G. EEG coherence in Alzheimer's disease. Electroencephalography and Clinical Neurophysiology. 1998;**106**(3):229-237

[94] Aftanas LI, Lotova NV, Koshkarov VI, Popov SA. Non-linear dynamical coupling between different brain areas during evoked emotions: An EEG investigation. Biological Psychology. 1998;**48**(2):121-138

[95] Gudmundsson S, Runarsson TP, Sigurdsson S, Eiriksdottir G, Johnsen K. Reliability of quantitative EEG features. Clinical Neurophysiology. 2007;**118**(10):2162-2171

[96] Fleck JI, Kuti J, Brown J, Mahon JR, Gayda-Chelder C. Frontal-posterior coherence and cognitive function in older adults. International Journal of Psychophysiology. 2016;**110**:217-230

[97] Adler G, Brassen S, Jajcevic A. EEG coherence in Alzheimer's dementia. Journal of Neural Transmission. 2003;**110**(9):1051-1058

[98] Leuchter AF, Newton TF, IANA C, Walter DO, Rosenberg-Thompson S, Lachenbruch PA. Changes in brain functional connectivity in Alzheimer-type and multi-infarct dementia. Brain. 1992;**115**(5):1543-1561

[99] Musaeus CS, Shafi MM, Santarnecchi E, Herman ST, Press DZ. Levetiracetam alters oscillatory connectivity in Alzheimer's disease. Journal of Alzheimer's Disease. 2017;**58**(4):1065-1076

[100] Moretti DV. Theta and alpha EEG frequency interplay in subjects with mild cognitive impairment: Evidence from EEG, MRI, and SPECT brain modifications. Frontiers in Aging Neuroscience. 2015;**7**:31

[101] Khan UA, Liu L, Provenzano FA, Berman DE, Profaci CP, Sloan R, et al. Molecular drivers and cortical spread of lateral entorhinal cortex dysfunction in preclinical Alzheimer's disease. Nature Neuroscience. 2014;**17**(2):304-311

[102] Babiloni C, Ferri R, Binetti G, Cassarino A, Dal Forno G, Ercolani M, et al. Fronto-parietal coupling of brain rhythms in mild cognitive impairment: A multicentric EEG study. Brain Research Bulletin. 2006;**69**(1):63-73

[103] Sonnen JA, Montine KS, Quinn JF, Kaye JA, Breitner JCS,

Montine TJ. Biomarkers for cognitive impairment and dementia in elderly people. Lancet Neurology. 2008;7(8):704-714

[104] Poil S-S, De Haan W, van der Flier WM, Mansvelder HD, Scheltens P, Linkenkaer-Hansen K. Integrative EEG biomarkers predict progression to Alzheimer's disease at the MCI stage. Frontiers in Aging Neuroscience. 2013;**5**:58

[105] Lista S, Garaci FG, Ewers M, Teipel S, Zetterberg H, Blennow K, et al. CSF Aβ1-42 combined with neuroimaging biomarkers in the early detection, diagnosis and prediction of Alzheimer's disease. Alzheimer's & Dementia. 2014;**10**(3):381-392

[106] Polikar R, Tilley C, Hillis B, Clark CM, Multimodal EEG. MRI and PET data fusion for Alzheimer's disease diagnosis. In: 2010 Annual International Conference of the IEEE Engineering in Medicine and Biology. IEEE. 2010. pp. 6058-6061

[107] Walhovd KB, Fjell AM, Brewer J, McEvoy LK, Fennema-Notestine C, Hagler DJ, et al. Combining MR imaging, positron-emission tomography, and CSF biomarkers in the diagnosis and prognosis of Alzheimer disease. American Journal of Neuroradiology. 2010;**31**(2):347-354

[108] Nielsen MS, Simonsen AH, Siersma V, Engedal K, Jelic V, Andersen BB, et al. Quantitative electroencephalography analyzed by statistical pattern recognition as a diagnostic and prognostic tool in mild cognitive impairment: Results from a Nordic multicenter cohort study. Dementia and Geriatric Cognitive Disorders Extra. 2018;**8**(3):426-438

[109] Houmani N, Vialatte F, Gallego-Jutglà E, Dreyfus G, Nguyen-Michel V-H, Mariani J, et al. Diagnosis of Alzheimer's disease with electroencephalography in a differential framework. PLoS One. 2018;**13**(3):e0193607

[110] Escudero J, Abásolo D, Hornero R, Espino P, López M. Analysis of electroencephalograms in Alzheimer's disease patients with multiscale entropy. Physiological Measurement. 2006;**27**(11):1091

[111] Zanin M, Zunino L, Rosso OA, Papo D. Permutation entropy and its main biomedical and econophysics applications: A review. Entropy. 2012;**14**(8):1553-1577

Chapter 5

Measurement and Evaluation of Brain Activity for Train Drivers Using Wearable NIRS

Hitoshi Tsunashima and Keita Aibara

Abstract

Human errors of train drivers may cause serious damage. Therefore, research on human error prevention has been conducted by many researchers. In this context, brain activity measurement of train drivers using near-infrared spectroscopy (NIRS) has been conducted to monitor the condition of train drivers. In this study, we developed a compact wireless wearable NIRS that can be used in natural environments. The wearable NIRS has been used to measure train drivers' brain function using a train driving simulator. Experimental results showed that brain activity of the dorsolateral prefrontal cortex (DLPFC) increased when the driver made braking operation. The experiment for train driving with an accidental event was carried out to evaluate the relation between drivers' attention and the brain activity. As a result, there was a difference in brain activity between with and without prior notice. Results showed that the increased attention of the train driver can be shown in the NIRS signal from the outer part of the prefrontal cortex.

Keywords: railway, train driver, human error, NIRS, condition monitoring

1. Introduction

Accidents due to human error while driving trains are rare but can cause severe and extensive damage when they do occur. Human error for train drivers refers to driving in an unusual condition, for example, when drowsy, exhausted, or in a hurry, which may lead to ignoring signals or speeding. Signaling systems such as automatic train protection (ATP) are used to prevent accidents caused by human error, yet not all accidents can be avoided even when these signaling systems are in place. Thus, research is being conducted to enable the monitoring of the status of train drivers, the early detection of abnormalities, and the prevention of accidents.

Functional near-infrared spectroscopy (fNIRS) was used to measure subjects' cerebral blood flow to investigate higher-order human brain function activity associated with cognition and attention while operating a vehicle [1, 2]. Lohani et al. provides a selective review of the psychophysiological measures that can be utilized to assess cognitive states in real-world driving environments [3]. Brain activity of train driver was measured using a 128-channel high-density electroencephalogram (EEG) while participants drove in a train driving simulator [4]. Kojima et al. analyzed the characteristics of brain activity measured in the prefrontal area with functional near-infrared spectroscopy (fNIRS) [5, 6]. However, there are many challenges to consider when applying these to the real world.

Conventional multichannel NIRS employs several cables to obtain readings. Furthermore, the probes placed on the head are heavy and are not suited for long-term monitoring. This has posed a problem for measuring brain activity in train drivers in real time. Recently, a lightweight and wireless wearable NIRS device was developed and has been used to measure brain function in car drivers. It is possible that this NIRS technology can also be applied to measure brain activity in train drivers.

While a wearable NIRS device places only a small burden on participants, can be used for assessment over long periods, and is applicable in the real world, it has fewer channels and cannot create a brain functional image, and thus is not suitable for the identification of activation areas. Meanwhile, multichannel NIRS device has several channels and is suitable for such identification, but places a burden on participants and is not a good match for measurement in the real world.

In this study, we first identified activation areas from a brain functional image using multichannel NIRS (Spectratech, OEG-16 [7]). We then measured brain activity in these areas using a wearable NIRS device (Astem, Hb131S [8]) and examined brain activity measurements from the channel signals, including the activation areas [9, 10].

This paper is an extended version of the published paper [11].

2. Principles of NIRS

NIRS is a method of measuring changes in hemoglobin concentration using near-infrared light (wavelength: 700–900 nm) which can penetrate deep into the living tissue. When nerve activity occurs, there is a local increase in blood flow and a change in hemoglobin concentration in the blood. It is possible to measure changes in concentration of oxygenated hemoglobin (oxy-Hb) and deoxygenated hemoglobin (deoxy-Hb) from the transmitted near-infrared light and attenuation of the diffused light [12, 13].

When measuring brain activity, near-infrared light is beamed from optical fibers placed on the surface of the head. This light reaches the surface of the brain while being absorbed and diffused by the scalp, cranium, and cerebrospinal fluid. The amount of transmitted light that returns to the surface of the head is then measured by the detector fibers, which can be used to calculate changes in the hemoglobin concentration on the surface of the brain.

Brain activity accounts for roughly 5% of local intracerebral oxygen consumption. In contrast, local intracerebral blood flow increases by 30–50%, far surpassing consumption. Consequently, an area in which there is brain activity will typically demonstrate an increase in oxy-Hb and a decrease in deoxy-Hb, and this change is seen in the surrounding brain regions as well. Thus, evaluating the amount of change in oxy-Hb makes it possible to understand the status of brain activity, and this feature is used by NIRS devices as the parameter which best reflects brain activation. In the present study, brain activity was analyzed using the amount of oxy-Hb change as the primary evaluation criteria.

NIRS also includes a method of measurement known as spatial resolved spectroscopy (SRS). SRS is a method of measuring oxygen saturation (StO2), which utilizes two detectors to measure two different optical path lengths. The wearable NIRS (Hb131S) used in the present study is equipped with SRS, thereby enabling the measurement of oxygen saturation, which is an effective indicator highly correlated with oxy-Hb and is not likely to be influenced by cutaneous blood flow. However, its sensitivity is low compared to oxy-Hb, and there are presently a few

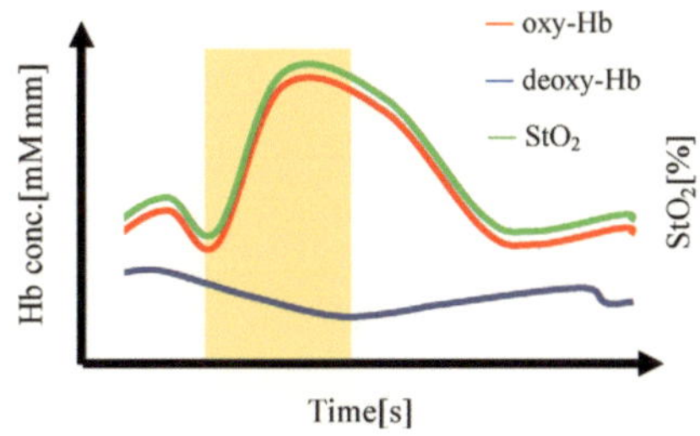

Figure 1.
Schematic of changes in hemoglobin concentration and oxygen saturation due to neural activity.

cases in which it is used as a primary evaluation index for brain activity. Therefore, deoxy-Hb and oxygen saturations were used as supplementary indicators to discern the existence of artifacts **Figure 1** shows a schematic of changes in hemoglobin concentration and oxygen saturation due to neural activity.

3. Method

3.1 Experimental equipment

In this experiment, brain activity was measured while driving a train using multichannel NIRS (OEG-16, Spectratech, 16ch, sampling rate: 0.66 s) and wearable NIRS (Hb131S, Astem, 4ch, sampling rate: 0.5 s). The multichannel NIRS was fitted so that the lowest row of channels was 40 mm from the base of the nose. The wearable NIRS was mounted so that 1ch corresponded to the vicinity of the multichannel NIRS 13ch.

Figure 2 shows the NIRS channels for OEG-16 and Hb131S, while **Figure 3** shows the Hb131S device. Fpz in 10–20 electrode system corresponds to the center of the NIRS cap. The Hb131S is completely wireless and lightweight, meaning that it can be used for measurement while driving a train without impeding operations. Furthermore, in addition to oxy-Hb and deoxy-Hb, which can be measured by normal NIRS, Hb131S is able to measure oxygen saturation.

The brain activity of train drivers was also measured using a train driving simulator which records the driving position, speed, acceleration, and handle notch position of master controller. **Figure 4** shows the experimental setup. **Figure 5** shows the handle notch position in the train driving simulator.

3.2 Station stopping task

Previous studies have confirmed increases in oxy-Hb in the DLPFC in areas in which drivers performed a deceleration operation (hereafter referred to as a braking area) with the goal of stopping [5, 6]. However, measurement using multichannel fNIRS (OMM-3000, Shimadzu, 42ch) places a large burden on participants and is difficult to use for long-term experiments. Therefore, we took measurements using a multichannel NIRS device (OEG-16, Spectratech, 16ch), which is able to measure more easily and has a smaller burden on participants when used to identify activation areas. Next, we considered whether measurement was possible with the smaller wearable NIRS which can be worn constantly, even in the real world.

Nine healthy men between the ages of 20 and 29 with an experience of driving a car, and who gave informed consent, participated in the station stopping task. Brain activity was measured during operation of the train driving simulator. In addition to the wearable NIRS Hb131S, measurement of the entire prefrontal area was

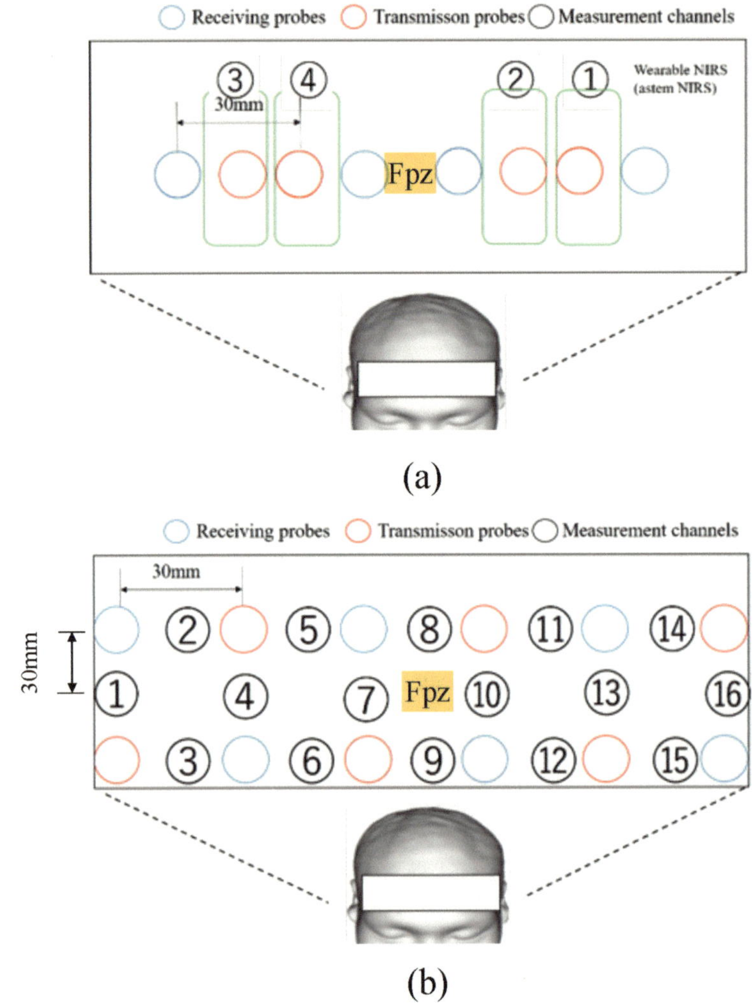

Figure 2.
Channel placement of NIRS (Hb131S and OEG16) [11]. (a) Wearable NIRS (Hb 131-S). (b) Multi-channel NIRS (OEG-16).

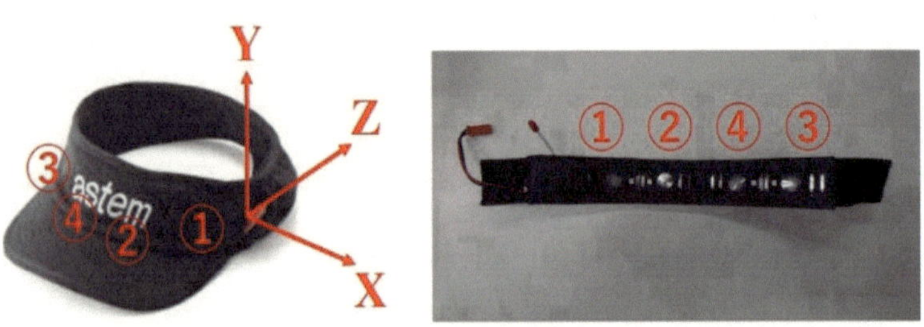

Figure 3.
Wearable NIRS: Hb131S [11].

conducted with the multichannel NIRS OEG-16 (16ch) for the station stopping task. We investigated whether the brain activity of train drivers could be measured using wearable NIRS technology through a comparison with the multichannel NIRS. In this study, we particularly focused on the 1ch in wearable NIRS and 13ch in multichannel NIRS, for which the channel positioning was the same.

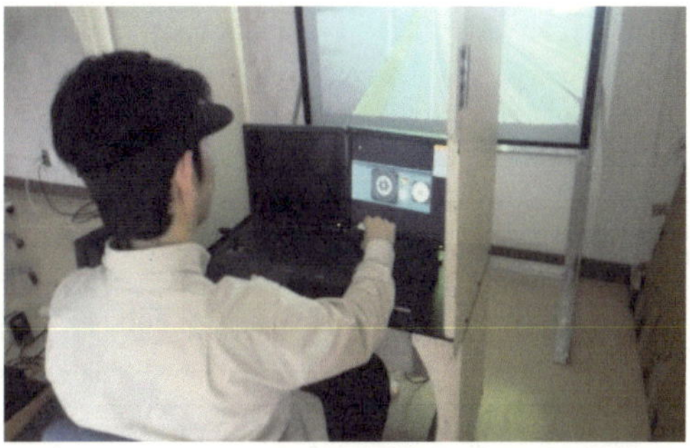

Figure 4.
Experimental setup using train driving simulator [11].

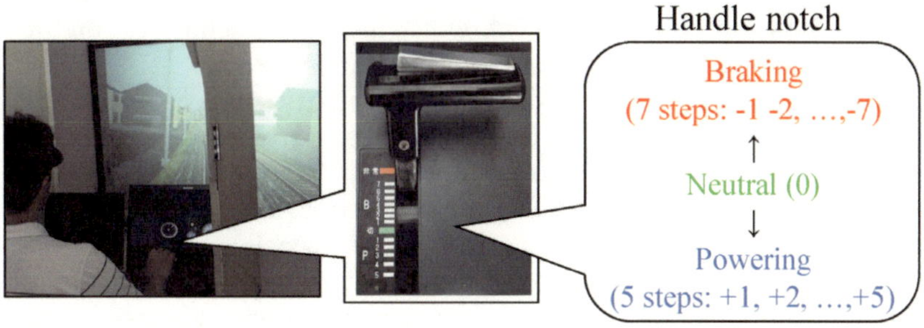

Figure 5.
Handle notch position in train driving simulator.

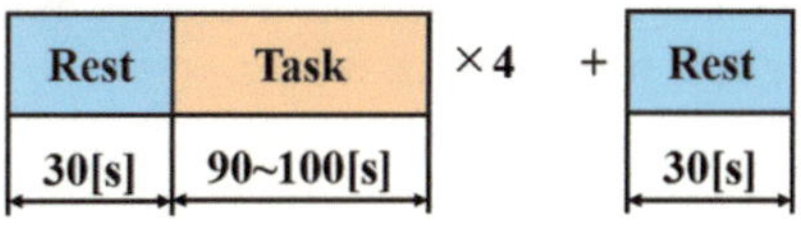

Figure 6.
Experimental design for train driving in normal condition [11].

The experimental design for the station stopping task is shown in **Figure 6**. For the rest of the periods during the station stopping task, participants rested for 30 s with their eyes closed. For the task periods, participants were instructed to drive from departure to designated stop, using only acceleration and deceleration and following the speed limit on a roughly 940 m section. A total of four trials were performed with one trial consisting of a rest period and a task period. The experiment was performed with a 2-day interval between the respective devices.

3.3 Obstacle avoidance task

Nakagawa et al. assessed the brain activity of drivers when they were shown an obstacle on the tracks in a train driving simulator using a 128-channel high-density EEG [4]. Similarly, in this study we showed participants an obstacle on the tracks and examined whether brain activity while driving could be evaluated from the cerebral blood flow. In particular, we evaluated whether drivers could appropriately process external environmental information while driving and maintain appropriate driving behaviors when abnormalities appeared (hereafter referred to as attentional state). Generally, individuals driving casually tend to have lower brain activity than those paying appropriate attention to the external environment.

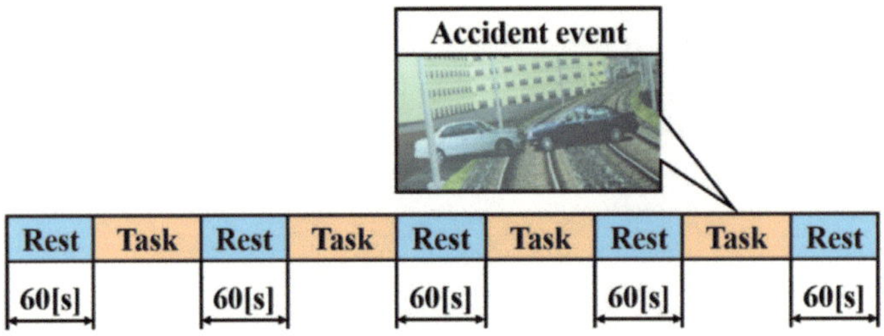

Figure 7.
Experimental design for train driving with an accidental event [11].

Eleven healthy men between the ages of 20 and 29 with an experience of driving a car, and who gave informed consent, participated in the obstacle avoidance task. We examined whether measurement of the attentional state was possible with wearable NIRS during an accident event, which involved placing a car on the tracks as the obstacle. The experimental design is shown in **Figure** 7.

The obstacle appearance was positioned such that participants needed to apply the emergency brake promptly when the obstacle was discovered in order to safely stop the train. One experiment in which the participant was not informed that an obstacle would appear and one in which they were informed were performed with each participant.

The experiment with no advanced notice of the obstacle was performed four times: the first three times were similar to the station stopping task, but on the fourth trial, the obstacle was presented. The experiment with advanced notice of the obstacle was performed next. For this experiment, participants were informed in advance that an obstacle would appear in one of the four trials and that they should promptly stop when the obstacle appeared during the task. In the task period of the obstacle avoidance task, a driving distance of approximately 1400 m between stations was selected. The rest periods lasted 60 s.

4. NIRS signal analysis method

NIRS signals include sounds from the body such as breathing and heartbeat. The signals also include trends across the entire experiment when measured over long periods. Therefore, signal processing was performed through multi-resolution analysis (MRA) [14, 15] using discrete wavelet transformation to extract only the brain activity components relevant to the research design [16].

Wavelet transform expresses the local shape of the waveform to be analyzed, $S(t)$, by shifting and dilating the waveform called the mother wavelet, $\psi(t)$, and then analyzes the waveform:

$$\int_{-\infty}^{+\infty} \psi(t)dt = 0 \tag{1}$$

which is dilated with a scale parameter a and translated by b as

$$\psi_{a,b}(t) = \frac{1}{\sqrt{a}}\psi\left(\frac{t-b}{a}\right). \tag{2}$$

The continuous wavelet transform of signal $S(t)$ is computed with $\psi_{a,b}(t)$ as

$$\tilde{S}(a,b) = \int_{-\infty}^{\infty} S(t)\psi_{a,b}^{*}(t)dt. \tag{3}$$

Here, ψ^* denotes the complex conjugate of ψ.

One can construct wavelets such that the dilated and translated function

$$\psi_{m,n}(t) = 2^{-m/2}\psi(2^{-m}t - n) \tag{4}$$

is an orthonormal base.

Discrete wavelet transform can be computed by

$$D_m = \int_{-\infty}^{\infty} S(t)\psi_{m,n}(t)dt. \tag{5}$$

In the continuous wavelet transform, information is duplicated, requiring many calculations. Discrete wavelet transform handles a smaller volume of information than continuous wavelet transform but is able to transform signals more efficiently. Furthermore, the use of an orthonormal base facilitates complete reconstruction of original signals without redundancy. The following section describes decomposition and reconstruction of signals using MRA.

MRA decomposes signals into a tree structure using the discrete wavelet transform. In the case of the object time series signals, $S(t)$, it decomposes the signals into an approximated component (low-frequency component) and multiple detailed components (high-frequency components).

A signal $S(t)$ can be expressed as follows by discrete wavelet transform using an orthonormal base $\psi_{m,n}$ as

$$S(t) = \sum_{n=-\infty}^{\infty} A_{m_0,n}\phi_{m_0,n}(t) + \sum_{m=-\infty}^{m_0}\sum_{n=-\infty}^{\infty} D_{m,n}\psi_{m,n}(t) \tag{6}$$

Here, $\phi_{m,n}(t)$ is the scaling function as defined by the following equation:

$$\phi_{m,n}(t) = 2^{-m/2}\phi(2^{-m}t - n). \tag{7}$$

The coefficient of the approximated component is calculated by

$$A_{m,n} = \int_{-\infty}^{\infty} S(t)\phi_{m,n}(t). \tag{8}$$

The detailed components of the signals on level m can be expressed by

$$d_m = \sum_{n=-\infty}^{\infty} D_{m,n}\psi_{m,n}(t) \tag{9}$$

Thus, the signal $S(t)$ can be expressed as

$$S(t) = a_{m_0} + \sum_{m=-\infty}^{m_0} d_m. \tag{10}$$

Task-related components can thus be reconstructed from detailed components d_m.

In the wavelet transform, the choice of a mother wavelet $\psi_{m,n}$ is important. We employed a *Daubechies* wavelet [17], which is an orthonormal base and is a compactly supported wavelet. The vanishing moments of the *Daubechies* wavelet can be changed by an index N. We decided to use a relatively high-order generating index, $N = 7$, based on the evaluation of reconstruction performance with the frequency of task and sampling rate of NIRS signal. One example of the analysis performed in this study is shown in **Figure 8**.

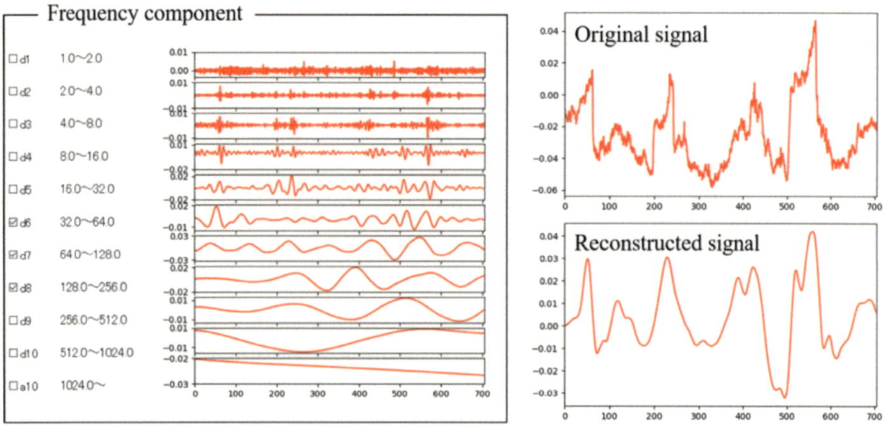

Figure 8.
Original signal and reconstructed signal using discrete wavelet transform [11].

Further, NIRS signals can be used to measure the relative amount of change in oxy-Hb and deoxy-Hb with the value at the start of measurement as the criteria. However, with the relative amount of change, comparisons between participants and statistical processing are difficult. As such, the data from oxy-Hb and deoxy-Hb that had undergone multi-resolution analyses were, respectively, Z-scored such that the mean would be 0 and the standard deviation would be 1, according to the following equation:

$$Z = \frac{X - \mu}{\sigma}. \tag{11}$$

Here, X represents the oxy-Hb or deoxy-Hb signal after reconstruction, while μ and σ refer to the mean and standard deviation, respectively.

The NIRS signals for each participant were resampled using linear interpolation as there was a variation in the periods between driving, starting, and stopping between the participants due to the nature of the experiment. Thereafter, time series data was converted to distance data, allowing it to be directly compared with the data obtained from the driving simulator. Furthermore, the arithmetic mean was calculated for the NIRS signals which had been converted into distance data for each participant and statistical processing performed.

5. Results

5.1 Station stopping task

Multi-resolution analysis and Z-scoring were performed for the multichannel NIRS data for each of the 9 participants (9 males, aged 21–27 years (mean $\pm$ SD $=$ 22.4 ± 1.7)).

Figure 9 shows the time course of 16 channels for OEG-16. It can be seen that the neuronal activity in the braking task increases in the wide area of the prefrontal cortex. This result is supposed to be due to the fact that all participants are not familiar enough with train driving.

The arithmetic mean ($n = 9$) results of the time series data converted into distance data for each trial are shown in **Figure 10**. **Figure 10(a)** shows the speed and notch data and **Figure 10(b)** the oxy-Hb and deoxy-Hb data of 13ch. **Figure 10**

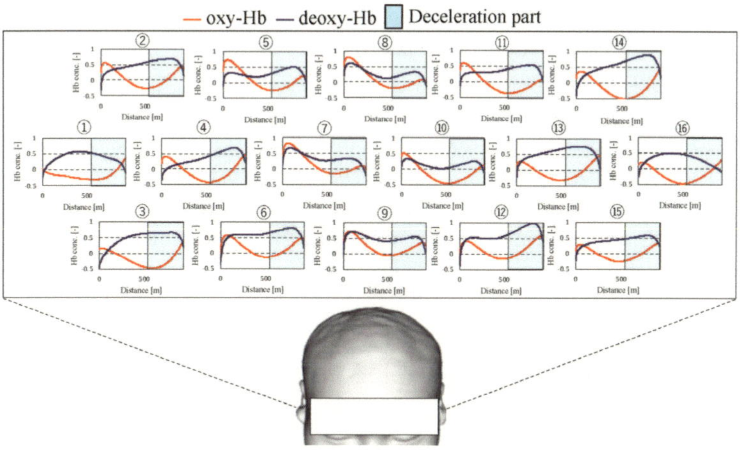

Figure 9.
Results of experiment for train driving in normal condition using OEG-16.

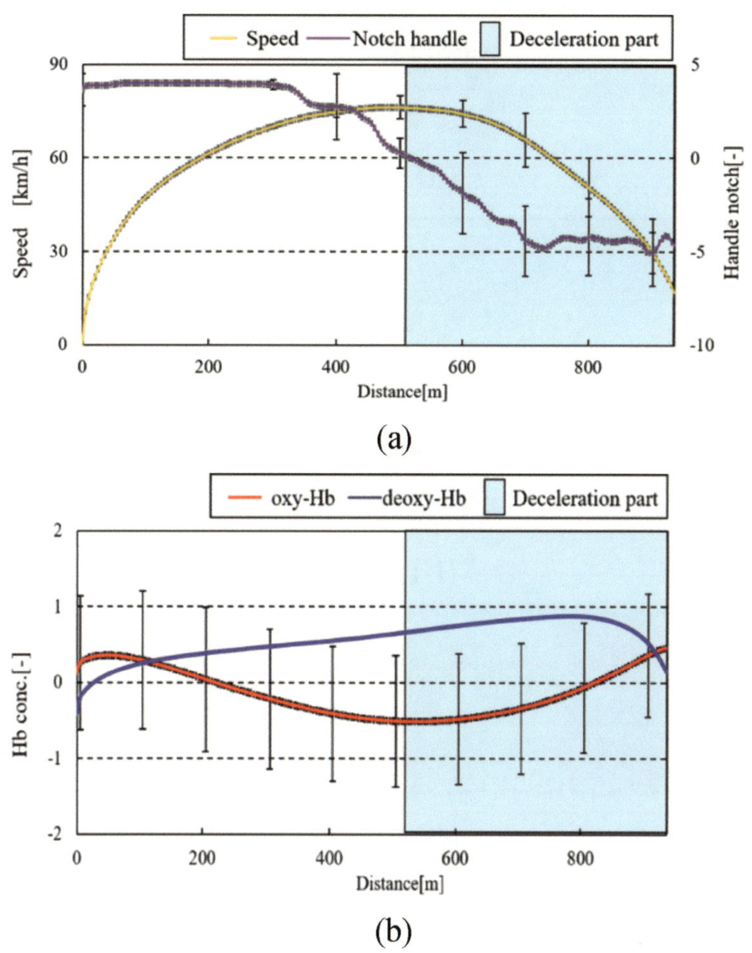

Figure 10.
Relation between speed, notch data, and oxy-Hb and deoxy-Hb of 13ch [11]. (a) Averaged result of speed and handle notch (n=9). (b)Averaged result of brain activity (n=9).

(a) demonstrates that the notch value became negative when the participant started braking in order to stop. Thus, **Figure 10(b)** confirmed that oxy-Hb signals tended to increase once braking had commenced.

This further designated the areas that should be focused on with wearable NIRS which has fewer channels. Therefore, brain functional images were created and evaluated for when participants first rested with their eyes closed during the experiment, during the acceleration operation (from the start of driving to the end of acceleration), and during the deceleration operation (from the deceleration start position to the stopping position), respectively. **Figure 11(a)** shows the functional brain image when resting with the eyes closed, **Figure 11(b)** during the acceleration operation, and **Figure 11(c)** during the deceleration operation.

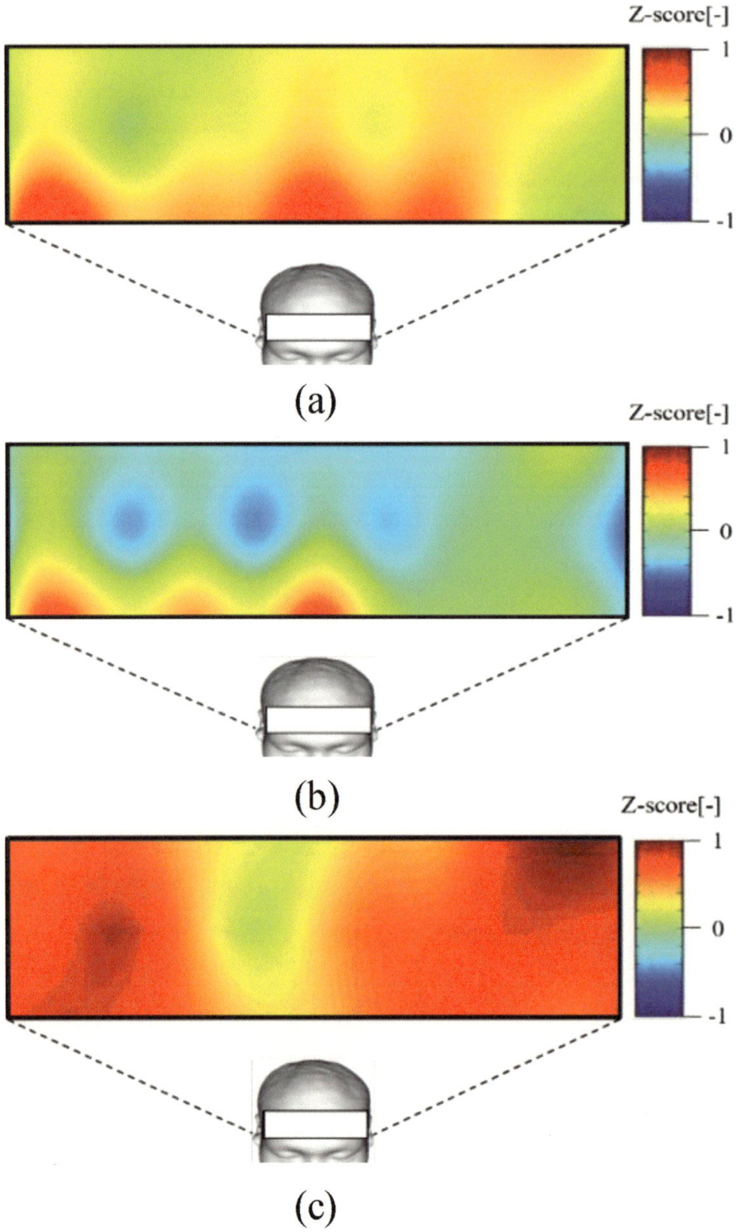

Figure 11.
Results of functional brain imaging (the bottom picture indicates the functional brain imaging during braking operation. It shows that outer portions of the prefrontal cortex are activated) [11]. (a) At rest. (b) During accelerating operation. (c) During braking operation.

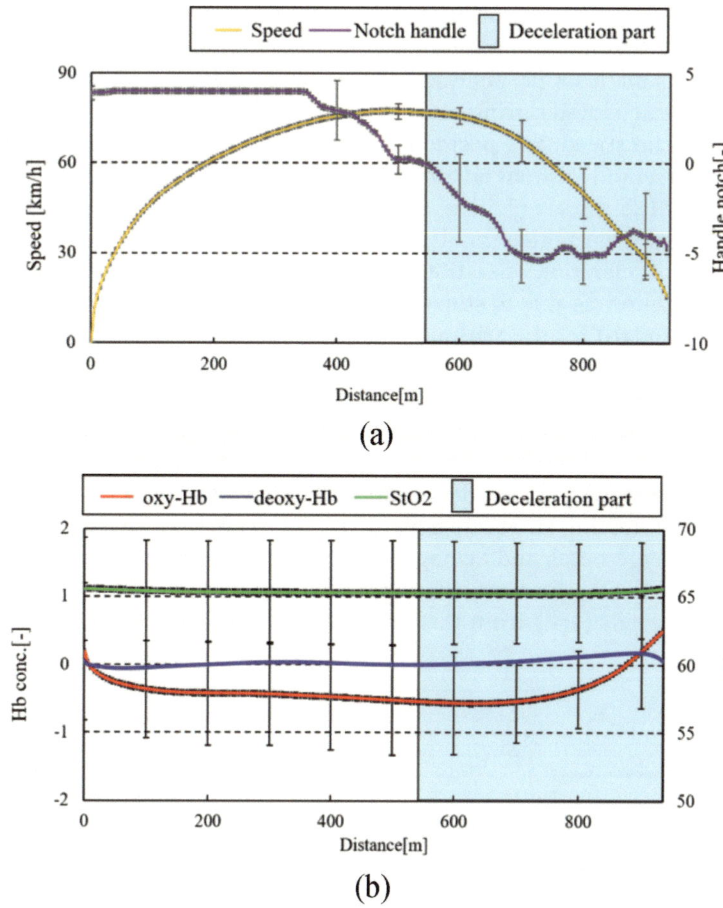

Figure 12.
Results of experiment for train driving in normal condition using wearable NIRS: Hb131S, 1ch (left outer portion) [11]. (a) Averaged result of speed and handle notch (n=9). (b)Averaged result of brain activity (n=9).

Brain activation in the dorsolateral areas was confirmed from the multichannel NIRS used in this study. Thus, for the wearable NIRS, analysis of the NIRS signals for each participant was performed with a focus on these areas. The left lateral area (1ch) of the wearable NIRS was analyzed in the same way as the multichannel NIRS. These results are shown in **Figure 12**. The arithmetic mean ($n = 9$) results for the notch data and speed for each distance are shown in **Figure 12(a)**. The arithmetic mean ($n = 9$) results for oxygen saturation and oxy-Hb and deoxy-Hb signals in the left lateral area for each distance are shown in **Figure 12(b)**.

In **Figure 12(a)**, the position at which the notch value becomes negative and deceleration begins was set as the deceleration start position. **Figure 12(b)** confirms that oxy-Hb and oxygen saturation tended to increase between the deceleration start position and stopping the train. The same trend was observed in the right lateral area. This confirms that the measurement of the drivers' brain activity using wearable NIRS was successful.

5.2 Obstacle avoidance task

Like the station stopping task, multi-resolution analysis and Z-scoring were performed for the wearable NIRS data for each of the 11 participants. Then the arithmetic mean ($n = 11$) was calculated for each trial. The same analysis was performed regardless of whether there was an advanced notice of the obstacle on the tracks. In this manuscript, analyses were performed for the lateral area that had been found to be activated during attention.

The notch, train speed, and position of the obstacle on the tracks for the trial in which it was presented without advanced notice are shown in **Figure 13(a)**. The time history of NIRS signals (1ch) is shown in **Figure 13(b)**. The obstacle car was presented without prior notice for all participants. As a result, it was not possible to quickly begin a deceleration operation and a collision with the obstacle occurred. The participant who was able to stop closest to the obstacle on the tracks (at 965 m) was used as a standard for the arithmetic mean.

Our finding that both oxy-Hb and StO2 decreased drastically when running a train under normal conditions is an indication that there are few driving operations required in such conditions, which cause a decline in concentration. We also confirmed that oxy-Hb and StO2 tended to increase when participants discovered an obstacle and performed a drastic deceleration. This trend implies that brain activity levels rose after detecting an obstacle on the tracks in order to be able to react to it.

Next, the average notch and average train speed for each participant in the trials with advanced notice of the obstacles appearance are shown in **Figure 14(a)**. The averaged NIRS signals (1ch) from this time are shown in **Figure 14(b)**. As with the

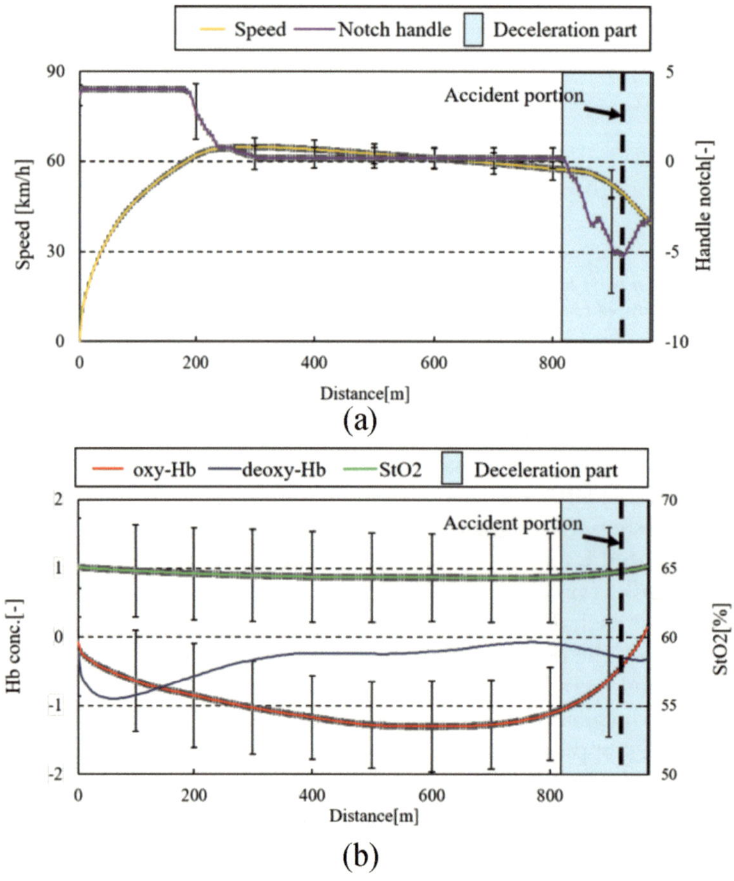

Figure 13.
Results of experiment for train driving with an accidental event using wearable NIRS: Hb131S, 1ch (left outer portion without prior notice). (a) Averaged result of speed and handle notch (n=11). (b)Averaged result of brain activity (n=11).

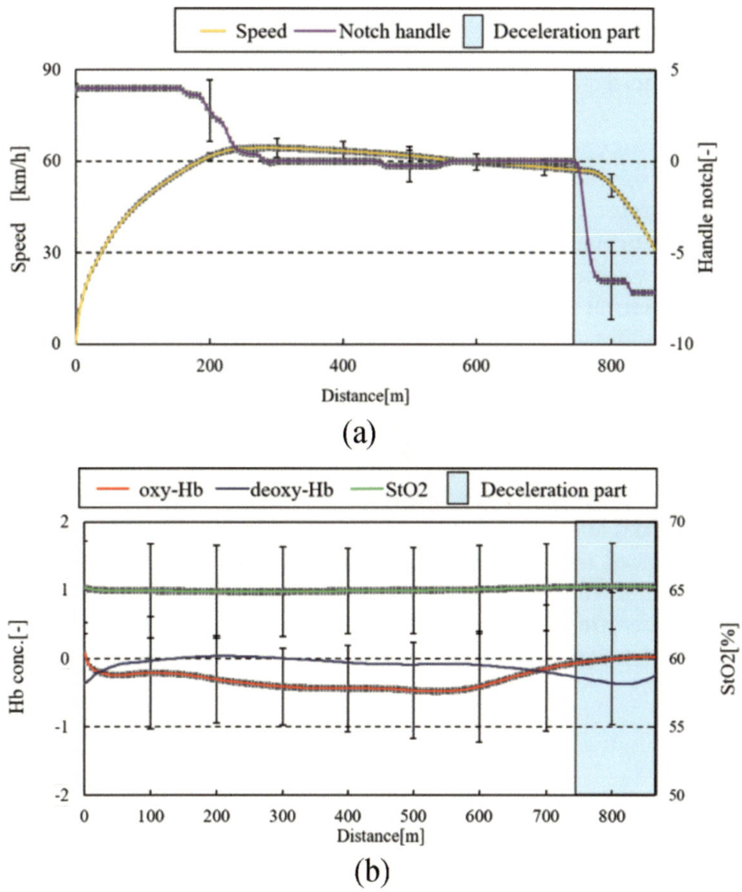

Figure 14.
Results of experiment for train driving with an accidental event wearable NIRS: Hb131S, 1ch (left outer portion with prior notice) [11]. (a) Averaged result of speed and handle notch (n=11). (b)Averaged result of brain activity (n=11).

experiment with advanced notice, the participant who stopped the nearest (865 m) was used as the standard for analysis.

When drivers were informed before the appearance of the obstacle, it can be concluded that they were focused and, therefore, were able to prevent a collision. Furthermore, the results of the measurement of brain activity in **Figure 13(b)** show that oxy-Hb and StO2 tended to decrease when accelerating. However, the change in oxy-Hb was lower than for **Figure 14(b)** in which there was advanced notice.

A previous study by Sakai and Kato confirmed that oxy-Hb value tends to increase when attention levels are high [18]. As such, it can be concluded that participants were driving with higher attention during the obstacle avoidance task. Furthermore, the measurement was regarded as successful and was not influenced by artifacts due to the high correlation confirmed between oxygen saturation and oxy-Hb.

6. Discussion

From the brain function images in **Figure 11**, no major changes in the brain are visible while at rest in normal driving task. When driving, there was a monotone decreasing trend in oxy-Hb only for the acceleration operation. The stopping operation during the deceleration operation was particularly complex. Thus, it is considered that there was bilateral activation of the lateral area due to learning the operation.

In a previous study, it was confirmed that bilateral activation of the dorsolateral prefrontal area is seen when learning an operation, while activation of the medial area is not, in a large-scale multichannel NIRS study of train drivers [5]. The increases of the neuronal activity in the dorsolateral prefrontal area can be related to the connection between the dorsolateral prefrontal area and the cerebellum. In the cerebellum, an internal model is constructed so that the brain manages driving effectively. The evidence of this fact has been shown by the experiment of train driving training for 6 months for a beginner driver. As the time goes by and driving performance improved, the neuronal activity in the dorsolateral prefrontal area decreased.

In the trial performed without advanced notice of the obstacle in the obstacle avoidance task, no participant was able to safely stop the train after discovering the obstacle. In contrast, all participants were able to stop directly before the obstacle when given advanced notice, and oxy-Hb was higher in this situation. This is likely because participants were on alert for the appearance of an obstacle, in addition to normal driving operations. This trend was seen in all participants, which demonstrates that the attentional state of train drivers can be evaluated using wearable NIRS.

7. Field test

We investigated whether the wearable NIRS (Hb131S) can be applied in real train operations. A field test was carried out at a train depot of a railway operator. The maximum speed of the test line was 15 km/h. **Figure 15** shows the train operation in the test line.

Measured raw data using wearable NIRS (Hb131S) was obtained from a train driver and is shown in **Figure 16**. The measured signals were processed to remove high-frequency noise, and the baseline correction between the tasks was performed. The signal processed oxy-Hb and handle notch position are shown in **Figure 17**.

It can be seen from **Figure 16** that oxy-Hb and StO2 increase at braking area. As we can see a good correlation between oxy-Hb and StO2, the measurement using wearable NIRS (Hb131S) was successful. It should be noted from **Figure 17** that

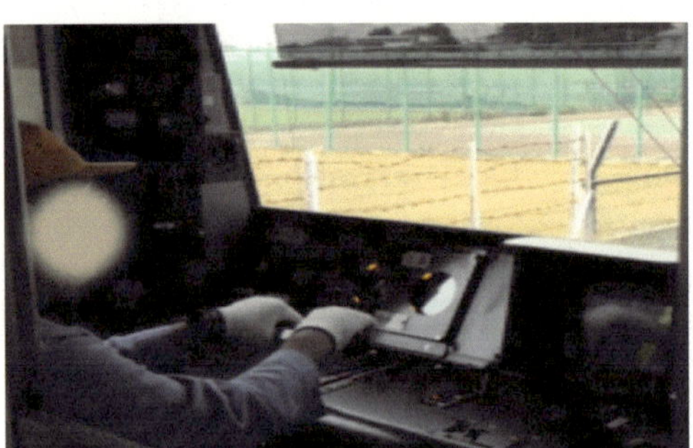

Figure 15.
Train operation in the test line.

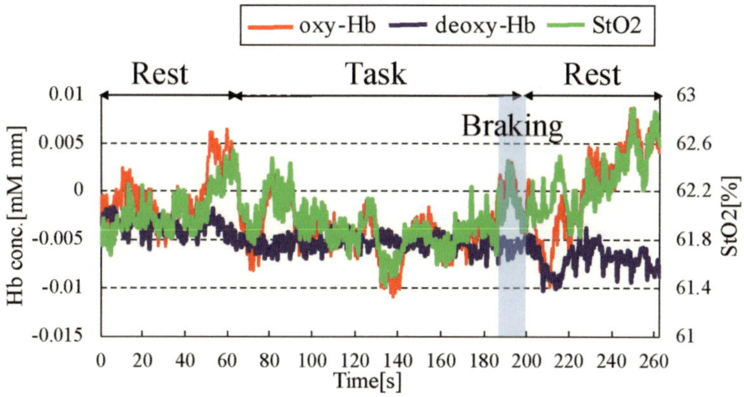

Figure 16.
Measurement data using wearable NIRS (Hb131S).

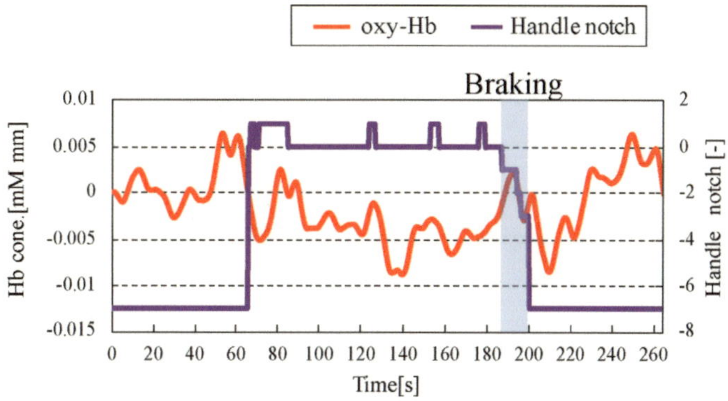

Figure 17.
Signal processed oxy-Hb and handle notch position in train operation.

oxy-Hb increases when the train driver operates the handle notch for train speed control particularly in the braking area.

8. Conclusion

This study aimed to examine the feasibility of monitoring the brain activity of train drivers using wearable NIRS. We investigated whether their brain activity could be measured using wearable NIRS, as well as whether their attentional states could be evaluated.

First, a general train-stopping task was carried out and multichannel NIRS compared to wearable NIRS. It was found that both NIRS devices confirmed elevation of oxy-Hb with a deceleration operation, which is consistent with earlier research. The wearable NIRS also confirmed elevation in oxy-Hb and StO2. Therefore, it was verified that the brain activity of train drivers can be measured using wearable NIRS.

Next, we carried out an obstacle avoidance task using wearable NIRS. Brain activity was measured in a condition with advanced notice of the obstacle and a condition without advanced notice to examine whether the attentional state could be evaluated. It was found that oxy-Hb was low prior to detecting an obstacle in the condition without notice. Oxy-Hb was higher in the condition with advanced notice. Therefore, it was proven possible to monitor attention levels from the brain activity of drivers using wearable NIRS.

Finally, we investigated whether the wearable NIRS can be applied in real train operations. A field test was carried out at a train depot of a railway operator. Field test results showed that the wearable NIRS can be applicable for measuring train drivers' brain function in real world.

Most of the related studies have been carried out in laboratories using a train driving simulator. The purpose of this study is to evaluate the applicability of wearable NIRS for train drivers in real world. As the wearable NIRS system has been recently developed, we need to collect many NIRS data in real train driving so that we can evaluate the train drivers' condition from NIRS data as our future work.

Acknowledgements

We are grateful to Ms. S. Makishima and Ms. M. Satozono for helping us with the field test and data analysis. We would like to thank Editage (www.editage.jp) for the English language editing.

Conflict of interest

The authors declare no conflict of interest.

Abbreviations

NIRS	near-infrared spectroscopy
DLPFC	dorsolateral prefrontal cortex
ATP	automatic train
oxy-Hb	oxygenated hemoglobin
deoxy-Hb	deoxygenated hemoglobin
StO2	oxygen saturation
fMRI	functional magnetic resonance imaging
fNIRS	functional near-infrared spectroscopy
SRS	spatial resolved spectroscopy
MRA	multi-resolution analysis

Author details

Hitoshi Tsunashima[1*†] and Keita Aibara[2†]

1 Department of Mechanical Engineering, College of Industrial Technology, Nihon University, Chiba, Japan

2 JEOL Ltd., Tokyo, Japan

*Address all correspondence to: tsunashima.hitoshi@nihon-u.ac.jp

† These authors are contributed equally.

References

[1] Tsunashima H, Yanagisawa K. Measurement of brain function of car driver using functional near-infrared spectroscopy (fNIRS). Computational Intelligence and Neuroscience. 2009; **2009**. Article ID 164958. DOI: 10.1155/2009/164958

[2] Shimizu T, Hirose S, Obara H, Yanagisawa K, Tsunashima H, Marumo Y, et al. Measurement of frontal cortex brain activity attributable to the driving workload and increased attention. SAE International Journal of Passenger Cars—Mechanical Systems. 2009;**2**(1):736-744. DOI: 10.4271/2009-01-0545

[3] Lohani M, Payne BR, Strayer DL. A review of psychophysiological measures to assess cognitive states in real-world driving. Frontiers in Human Neuroscience. 2019;**13**:57. DOI: 10.3389/fnhum.2019.00057

[4] Nakagawa C, Akiu N, Yoshie S, Kojima T, Watanabe T, Suzuki A. Basic study on assessment of state of the drivers based on physiological indices. RTRI Report (in Japanese). 2019;**33**(1)

[5] Kojima T, Tsunashima H, Shiozawa T, Takada H, Sakai T. Measurement of train driver's brain activity by functional near-infrared spectroscopy (fNIRS). Optical and Quantum Electronics. 2005;**37**(13-15). DOI: 10.1007/s11082-005-4202-9

[6] Kojima T, Tsunashima H, Shiozawa T. Measurement of train driver's brain activity by functional near-infrared spectroscopy (fNIRS). In: Computers in Railways X. WIT Press; 2006:245-254

[7] Spectratech, OEG-16. Available from: http://www.spectratech.co.jp/En/product/productOeg16En.html

[8] AstemHb131S. Available from: http://www.astem-en.com/nirs-devices/

[9] Jöbsis FF. Noninvasive, infrared monitoring of cerebral and myocardial oxygen sufficiency and circulatory parameters. Science. 23 December 1977: **198**(4323):1264-1267. DOI: 10.1126/science.929199

[10] Fukuda M. Near-infrared spectroscopy as a clinically available laboratory test for diagnosis and treatment of psychiatric disorders. MEDIX (in Japanese). 2003

[11] Aibara K, Shimizu R, Takanaka R, Tsunashima H. Measurement and evaluation of brain activity for train drivers using wearable NIRS. Transactions of the JSME (in Japanese). 2019;**85**(871). DOI: 10.1299/transjsme.18-00116

[12] Hoshi Y, Kobayashi N, Tamura M. Interpretation of nearinfrared spectroscopy signals, a study with a newly developed perfused rat brain model. Journal of Applied Physiology. 2001;**90**(5):1657-1662

[13] Tamura M. Functional near-infrared spectoroscopy. Advances in Neurological Sciences, Series C. 2003; **47**(6):891-901

[14] Mallat S. A theory for multiresolution signal decomposition: The wavelet representation. IEEE Transactions on Pattern Recognition and Machine Intelligence. 1989;**11**(7): 674-693

[15] Mallat S. A Wavelet Tour of Signal Processing. Academic Press. ISBN 978-0124666061

[16] Tsunashima H, Kazuki Yanagisawa K, Iwadate M. Measurement of brain function using near-infrared spectroscopy (NIRS). In: Bright P, editor. Neuroimaging. IntechOpen; 2012. pp. 75-98. DOI: 10.5772/22854.ch4

[17] Daubechies I. Ten Lectures on Wavelets: Society for Industrial and Applied Mathematics. CBMS-NSF Regional Conference Series in Applied Mathematics. SIAM. Vol. 61. 1992. ISBN: 0898712742, 9780898712742

[18] Sakai H, Kato T. A change of the blood hemoglobin density in a prefrontal area at the time of attention control task enforcement: Examination with "Kanahiroi" multi-cancellation test. Health Science (in Japanese). Kyoto University; 2006;**3**:7-15. DOI: 10.14989/48834

Section 3

Clinical Trials Network

Chapter 6

Imaging and Neuro-Oncology Clinical Trials of the National Clinical Trials Network (NCTN)

Thomas J. FitzGerald, Maryann Bishop-Jodoin, Fran Laurie, Richard Hanusik, Matthew Iandoli, Kathryn Karolczuk, Sandra Kessel, Fred Prior, Joel Saltz, Ashish Sharma, Michael Knopp, Mark Rosen, Ying Xiao, David Followill, Jeff Michalski, M. Giulia Cicchetti and Janaki Moni

Abstract

Imaging in neuro-oncology clinical trials can be used to validate patient eligibility, stage at presentation, response to therapy, and radiation therapy. A number of National Clinical Trials Network trials illustrating this are presented. Through the Imaging and Radiation Oncology Core's quality assurance processes for data acquisition and review, there are uniform data and imaging sets for review. Once the trial endpoints have been analyzed and published, the clinical trial information including pathology, imaging, and radiation therapy objects can be moved to a public archive for use by investigators interested in translational science and the application of new informatics tools for trial analysis.

Keywords: imaging, radiation therapy, clinical trials, targeted therapy, cancer treatment

1. Introduction

Over the past three decades, imaging has become an important component of successful execution and completion of clinical trials for the National Clinical Trials Network (NCTN) of the National Cancer Institute (NCI). Imaging used in clinical trials serves as a biomarker to validate patient eligibility, stage at presentation, and response to therapy. Once archived, imaging becomes an inexhaustible resource to compare response to historical standards and validate tools for analysis of trial outcome. The quality of the imaging archive is essential to the NCTN and clinical translational investigators. Data acquisition and management quality assurance processes are imbedded in trials to ensure that the required trial-specific imaging is collected and organized according to standards. Modern neuro-oncology clinical trials use anatomic and metabolic imaging with sequences and quality standards specific to each clinical trial charter. In this manuscript, we will review the history of imaging in clinical trials and the current status of neuro-oncology imaging in the NCTN. Future initiatives and vision for image integration with subject-specific biomarkers in neuro-oncology trials will be presented.

2. History of imaging in the NCTN

There is a rich history of clinical trial development within the NCI's clinical trials network. In the early development of the cooperative group clinical trials program, emphasis was placed on clinical protocols with onsite physician assessment of response and site-associated application of radiation therapy treatment objects. Even in trials that required radiation therapy, little information was made available to the clinical trial investigators concerning the abnormality defined on imaging, choice of area treated with radiation therapy, and dose to target. Because computational algorithms for dose calculation were varied and driven in part by individual institutional structure and process, the initial quality assurance processes in radiation oncology placed emphasis on creating uniformity of these processes with less emphasis on imaging and the application of imaging to target. By 1972, committees in the cooperative groups identified mechanisms to acquire information about targets treated. This included review of radiation therapy kilovoltage (kV) simulation images and megavoltage (MV) therapy portal images to confirm that what was intended to be delivered was treated. The trial-required information had to be forwarded to quality assurance centers as hard copies, where it was reviewed for trial compliance. These quality assurance reviews were performed largely in retrospect, as trials reached closure, due to the cumbersome data submission process. As the data acquisition processes became more familiar to investigators, efforts were made to review hard copy objects early in the radiation treatment process to ensure that the treatment plan met study guidelines [1, 2].

By 1980, three-dimensional volumetric radiation therapy treatment planning was being introduced to clinical trials as well as using electronic media to transmit data. The initial effort in volumetric electronic data collected placed emphasis on prostate carcinoma; however, the importance of imaging in the quality review process for radiation oncology began to become more visible and prominent in multiple disease sites including lymphoma. In the Pediatric Oncology Group (POG) protocol 8725, the objectives of the study were to randomize the role of radiation therapy in what would be called intermediate to advanced stage subjects by modern standards. The subjects received eight cycles of hybrid chemotherapy and are then randomized to receive radiation therapy to all initial sites of disease or complete their care without radiation. In the initial publication of the trial, there was no added benefit to the addition of radiation therapy to this population of subjects. However, in a subset analysis, those subjects that were treated by study standards and had all sites of disease treated at presentation had a 10% statistically significant disease-free survival benefit [3]. In other words, excluding sites of original disease was detrimental to outcome. Imaging was essential to this interpretation as well as the application of diagnostic imaging to radiation therapy treatment execution. This was one of the first trials that acquired imaging both at baseline and at closure of chemotherapy as radiation therapy targets had to be designed to imaging parameters and sites of disease at presentation with response-adapted blocking applied to mediastinal disease. Without imaging submitted for trial review, this interpretation could not be made. Today the partnership between imaging and radiation therapy is synergistic, and radiation therapy is fully dependent on image-guided platforms for modern patient care [4, 5].

The next iteration of Hodgkin lymphoma studies evaluated both early stage and intermediate stage subjects with response-adapted treatment. Because of the

DOI: http://dx.doi.org/10.5772/intechopen.89065

non-compliant radiation therapy issues in POG 8725, the imaging and the radiation therapy treatment objects, as based on the disease at presentation, were reviewed by the Quality Assurance Review Center (QARC) before the start of radiation therapy. Pre- and post-chemotherapy imaging were reviewed to assess radiation therapy compliance. Compliance to radiation therapy was achieved; however, retrospective analysis of imaging response to chemotherapy demonstrated that central review disagreed with site assessment on 50% of cases [6]. Therefore, in the next iteration of trials evaluating intermediate risk subjects, imaging and radiation therapy objects were reviewed through a central mechanism in real-time pre-therapy, post two cycles of chemotherapy, post all chemotherapy, and pre-radiation therapy to ensure that response assessment was consistent with study objectives and radiation therapy was applied uniformly throughout the trial. Children's Oncology Group (COG) trial AHOD0331 accrued more than 1700 subjects and demonstrated that both anatomic and metabolic imaging and radiation therapy objects could be reviewed in an electronic format in real time at multiple study endpoints and permit adaptive therapy based on response to treatment. This infrastructure provided a platform to emphasize the importance of imaging in clinical trials as well as a mechanism to use imaging as a validation vehicle for successful execution of clinical trials. Because imaging can be simultaneously reviewed by multiple individuals including site and study investigators in real time, consensus between investigators could reach closure in a timely manner. Subject-specific issues and optimization of clinical trial management were addressed in a uniform manner and as early as the subject was enrolled on the trial [5, 7, 8].

The informatics platform quickly matured to support imaging in all pediatric and adult oncology radiology and radiation therapy disease service areas including neuro-oncology with real-time review of imaging objects to ensure study compliance. Protocols for standard risk medulloblastoma originating in the posterior fossa require no more than 1.5 cm^3 of residual disease and no evidence of disease on spine imaging at presentation. These objects are reviewed immediately in real time prior to subject entry onto study to ensure that the subject has entered onto the appropriate study and staged in a manner consistent with study objectives. Studies have confirmed that high-risk medulloblastoma patients unintentionally entered on low-risk studies have a significantly worse outcome, thus obfuscating interpretation of the study when evaluated on an intent to treat basis [9]. Completeness of resection is reviewed in real time for patients with ependymoma to ensure that the sequence of care including second surgical procedure as required by study is consistent with study guidelines. These changes in process serve to improve the quality of the study and are adjudicated by imaging. Imaging is identified as an essential component to successful clinical trial execution and by 1996 became well positioned to be recognized as a strong and independent discipline in the national clinical trials effort [3].

In 1997, Robert Wittes, MD, was the director of the Cancer Treatment Evaluation Program (CTEP) and recognized the need to develop an imaging program in clinical trials to function at an enterprise level. The NCI established a cancer imaging program under the direction of Daniel Sullivan, MD. In September of 1998, the American College of Radiology Imaging Network (ACRIN) was established under the direction of Bruce Hillman, MD, and Constantine Gatsonis, PhD. ACRIN had significant initial success managing important cancer screening trials including the digital mammography imaging screening trial (DMIST) and the National Lung Screening Trial (NLST). ACRIN has significant influence in credentialing institutions for imaging clinical trial participation and data management of clinical trials in all oncology disease areas including neuro-oncology imaging. ACRIN also participates in clinical trials including cardiology, interventional radiology, and advanced technology neurological imaging in non-oncology-related areas serving to further expand their portfolio and scope of service. ACRIN has partnered with the Eastern Clinical Oncology Group (ECOG) to bring its robust imaging infrastructure to support activities in a strong cooperative group with multiple disease committees. As ECOG-ACRIN, a strong standard is established for clinical trial interactions between clinical scientists and imaging partners. The imaging information for ECOG-ACRIN is managed by the Imaging and Radiation Oncology Core office in Philadelphia (IROC Philadelphia).

Of equal strength is the Wright Center of Innovation in Biomedical Imaging at the Ohio State University. Under the direction of Michael Knopp, MD, PhD, the Wright Center has obtained several major grant awards including a Frontier grant from the state of Ohio and a biomedical research and technology transfer award. The center houses expertise in microimaging, molecular imaging, animal imaging, as well as advanced technology imaging to support clinical trial processes. The Wright Center supports all the imaging needs including data management and real-time case review for the Alliance and SWOG clinical trial groups including significant expertise in neuroimaging and case evaluation. The Wright Center has developed processes to track compliance to anatomic and metabolic images acquired for clinical trials. The neuro-oncology committees are exceptionally strong, and neuro-oncology and neuroimaging are prominent disease-oriented committees in these important groups. Lawrence Schwartz, MD directs the imaging committees for Alliance and SWOG and works in close collaboration with the Wright Center for clinical trial execution. The office managing imaging information at the Wright Center for Alliance and SWOG is the Imaging and Radiation Oncology Core at Ohio (IROC Ohio).

Formerly known as Quality Assurance Review Center (QARC), the Imaging and Radiation Oncology Core center in Rhode Island (IROC RI) is responsible for imaging needs in COG. The imaging committee in COG became a formal discipline committee at the time of the merger between the Pediatric Oncology Group (POG) and Children's Cancer Group (CCG). QARC worked with committee members to establish an informatics infrastructure required for digital image transfer. This was accomplished by Keith White, MD, in collaboration with the information technology group at QARC. Data acquisition tools were applied to the process that he used to acquire and display images for tumor board at his home institution. The acquisition process is now synergistic with the data acquisition for radiation therapy treatment objects, and these can now be displayed in the IROC RI database for remote review of objects in a side-by-side manner by site and study investigators. Clinical trial investigators in all clinical disciplines including imaging and radiation oncology can review study objects in a harmonized and single-session manner. Because clinical trials require real-time review of objects for response assessment-adaptive clinical trials and the subsequent application of radiation therapy, each month, there are hundreds of study investigator logins to assure adaptive trial design is met and response/disease progression is noted and assessed in a uniform manner (**Figure 1**). Neuro-oncology imaging is essential to mission for COG as brain tumors comprise 25% of pediatric oncology. It is important that all image datasets including pre-/post-surgery/therapy and outcome imaging be available for review on a real-time basis as needed. The image library housed at IROC RI is the largest collection of pediatric oncology imaging in the world on patients treated on clinical trials with a complete portfolio of images on neuro-oncology patients treated on clinical protocols. The IROC Houston office (formerly the Radiological Physics Center (RPC)) works with all radiation oncology discipline committees of the NCTN and is the central resource for credentialing institutions for participation in clinical trials managed through the NCTN.

IROC is a single grant with overarching administrative structure to four grant offices in Houston TX, Columbus OH, Philadelphia PA, and Lincoln RI. Administrative support is provided by the American College of Radiology (ACR). IROC provides credentialing and data management for the NCTN in imaging and radiation oncology clinical trial participation (**Figure 2**). All offices that provide imaging data management services are involved in neuroimaging in NCTN clinical trials. The offices all collaborate with NCTN investigators to write uniform guidelines into all clinical trials involving the central nervous system (CNS) to ensure optimal clinical trial management and uniform response assessment. Modern guidelines include sequence acquisition requirements, slice thickness, and other acquisition parameters, which are written into every protocol by study investigators and IROC. The guidelines support both pediatric and adult clinical trials in neuro-oncology.

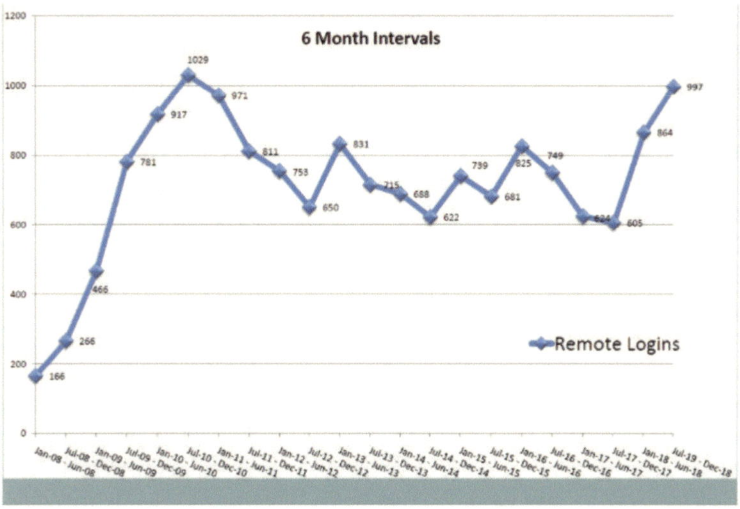

Figure 1.
Number of remote NCTN reviewer logins to terminal servers 2007–2019. Image courtesy of QARC.

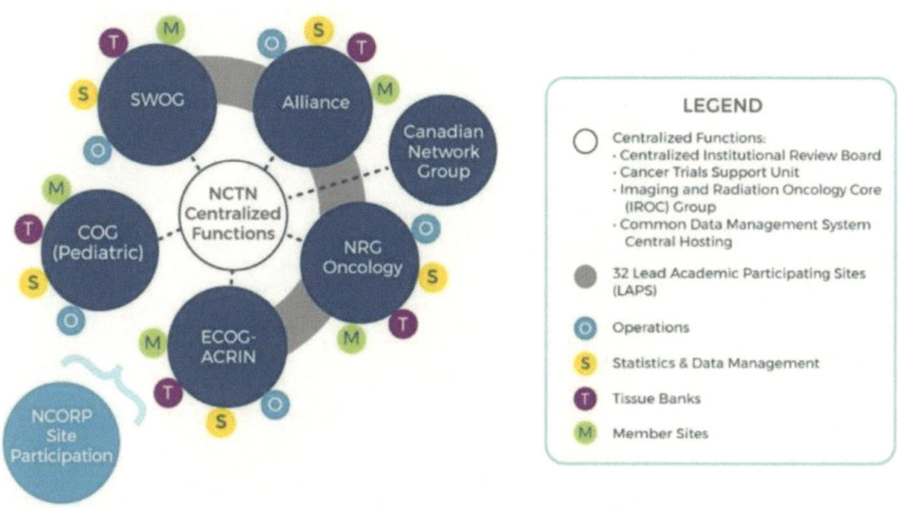

Figure 2.
NCI National Clinical Trials Network Structure. IROC is within the NCTN centralized functions. Image courtesy of the National Cancer Institute.

3. The importance of imaging applications in radiation therapy

Imaging platforms have become essential to daily operation in radiation oncology. From initial assessment of imaging for target definition to daily treatment alignment with cone beam computed tomography (CT), imaging has become an essential component of the infrastructure to successful delivery of daily radiation therapy. Imaging has likewise become essential for credentialing institutions to participate in clinical trials involving the CNS including the use of phantom technology for CNS magnetic resonance imaging (MRI) and application of radiation therapy. In an early iteration of the use of imaging as a credentialing vehicle, institutions received a planning image with a right temporal target and were asked to develop a therapy plan using a vertex field. This evaluated the ability of the institution to use three-dimensional modeling for therapy planning. Most radiation therapy planning systems are based on CT obtained in the therapy position with the appropriate immobilization device. CT, however, has significant limitations in defining targets for radiation therapy for lesions in the CNS. For clinical trials involving stereotactic radiosurgery (SRS), a credentialing vehicle was constructed where an institution would receive a planning CT with SRS coordinates. The target lesion was not visible on CT. An MR with a visible single lesion was provided, and the institution had to fuse the images into the site radiation planning system and provide x, y, and z coordinates for a stereotactic procedure [10]. The high-resolution and reality imaging registration processing evaluates both fusion tools and treatment planning capabilities. Anthropomorphic phantom tools have been developed by the IROC Houston office that require image validation for target definition as part of the credentialing process. This cross-validation has been essential for both documentation of image and assessment of the site computational planning algorithms (**Figure 3**).

Because tumors of the central nervous system are better defined with advanced technology imaging including advanced MR sequences and spectroscopy, fusion of images in treatment planning CT is a great resource and significantly improves target definition and patient care. In current NCTN protocols, advanced MR sequences are integrated with new positron emission tomography tracers including amino acid imaging and spectroscopy to create multiple target volumes treated with dose painting to areas of sequence abnormality. This is of increasing importance. Historically, neurosurgeons would remove regions of contrast enhancement seen on

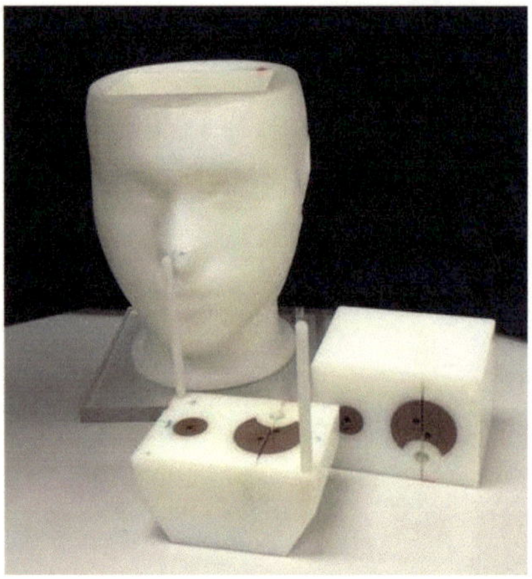

Figure 3.
Phantom tool developed by IROC Houston used in the RT site credentialing process. 1520 RT sites have passed at least one irradiation of this phantom. Image courtesy of IROC Houston.

CT and limited MR signal changes. Radiation oncologists, even on study, often treat the surgical resection site with a margin. With more primitive anatomical imaging, radiation oncologists performed poorly in defining the target volume of interest and may have not treated the entire tumor volume at risk on historical studies. New imaging models including amino acid imaging are demonstrating regions of tumor proliferation and tumor DNA synthesis which have been less visible and as a result, undertreated by radiation oncology. In primary brain patients, Investigators have confirmed that disease can reside in regions of FLAIR enhancement, thus influencing the choice of radiation therapy field placement. Spectroscopy may likewise be helpful moving forward in better defining targets at risk, and this is currently under evaluation with dose painting clinical trials in glioblastoma. Several papers have interesting reviews evaluating patterns of failure [11, 12]. In patients whose disease abutted central structures including the corpus callosum, failure patterns followed major nerve pathways into the contralateral hemisphere. If the anatomic and metabolic tumor target could be more optimally defined at presentation, we would potentially treat the patient more effectively with radiation therapy, hence possibly improving outcomes, as there is a high index of suspicion that simply targeting the region of contrast enhancement with margin may be insufficient for radiation therapy. Current protocols are using advanced imaging tools for target definition and dose painting. The volumes treated between T2 and FLAIR imaging were very different. Accordingly, the radiation fields are larger than targeting areas of contrast enhancement, and it will be important to monitor toxicity and pattern of failure with biomarker analysis [13].

Outcome imaging is important in clinical trials and often requires central review of imaging objects to provide consistent interpretation of treatment effect and disease progression. This is essential as often changes seen on MRI post-therapy can mimic disease progression. The NCTN pediatric and adult oncology databases include subjects with disease of the CNS including spine. These databases store imaging at presentation, pre- and post-surgery, radiation therapy treatment objects, and post-therapy. Because these images were obtained on study, the sequences and time points of data acquisition post-therapy are uniform in acquisition. These become optimal datasets for the development of machine learning and artificial intelligence tools to better evaluate this dilemma. The databases are linked to outcome through the statistical centers of each of the network groups and therefore are an invaluable resource to the field of neuro-oncology [9].

4. Current portfolio for neuro-oncology analysis in IROC

The Imaging and Radiation Oncology Core (IROC) houses all diagnostic imaging and radiation therapy treatment objects on subjects treated on clinical trials for the NCTN. The IROC office in RI works with the Children's Oncology Group (COG) and houses objects on subjects treated on clinical trials for more than 35 years. IROC RI also houses radiation therapy treatment objects for SWOG, Alliance, and ECOG-ACRIN. Trials include management of standard and high-risk medulloblastoma, ependymoma, primitive neuroendocrine tumors, germ cell tumors, and low-/high-grade glioma. Trials have studied the addition of chemotherapy to radiation therapy in multiple disease sites, sequence of management, and drug X-ray dose titration/augmentation. Modern protocols have applied adaptive strategies to titrate therapy to younger population, limit radiation boost dose to lesions that undergo gross tumor resection, and alter therapeutic application to medulloblastoma relative to tumor gene expression profiles. The IROC Ohio office manages neuro-oncology imaging for SWOG and Alliance. The Alliance group has an exceptionally strong neuro-oncology committee with primary emphasis in developing clinical trials for adult glioblastoma including studies directed to new modalities of care integrated with modern genomics and gene expression profiles. The IROC office in Philadelphia integrates the imaging strengths of imaging with ACRIN and the radiation oncology strengths of NRG (former NSABP, RTOG, and GOG). The emphasis of these groups is in the application of modern radiation oncology technology coupled with biomarker-driven applied chemo/targeted therapy for adult glioblastoma. Currently, IROC RI houses information on 24 protocols with datasets on over 3000 patients including imaging at presentation, post-therapy, relapse, and radiation therapy treatment objects for pattern of failure analysis. These include studies on primitive neuroectodermal disease, germ cell disease, high-/low-grade glioma, atypical rhabdoid lesion, medulloblastoma, and ependymoma. IROC Ohio houses images on more than 2000 patients treated for glioblastoma as well as images on protocols treating meningioma. The protocols include patients treated with vaccine therapy, antiangiogenetic therapy, and poly ADP ribose polymerase (PARP) inhibitors in patients with O[6]-methylguanine-DNA methyltransferase (MGMT) promotor hypermethylation as well as studies evaluating anaplastic and/or low-grade glioma treated with adjuvant PCV chemotherapy including those with 1p/19q co-deletions. IROC Philadelphia manages a similar volume of patients on study treated for glioblastoma with emphasis on radiation therapy target definition and technique. Each of the IROC centers manages advanced technology-driven imaging for radiosurgery for central nervous system metastatic disease. Neuro-oncology protocols managed by each of the IROC offices and available datasets are used for secondary clinical translational research objectives.

In the next generation of translational research for neuro-oncology, integration of biomarkers including genomics and applied gene expression profiles will need to be coupled with radiomics integrated with radiation therapy treatment plans. Ex vivo tissue unfortunately is an exhaustible resource and needs to be preserved for unanticipated biomarker evaluation in addition to current portfolios. Digital quantitative pathology will play an important role to integrate established and validated non-imaging biomarkers and biomarker processes with microscopy imaging signals to better predict outcome. Saltz and colleagues have integrated pathology biomarkers with imaging signals. Erickson and colleagues have identified radiomic signatures in glioblastoma patients that indicate and predict gene expression and methylation. Harmonization of this effort at an enterprise level will be the next step in developing improved tools for translational science [14–19].

5. The Cancer Imaging Archive (TCIA)

The Cancer Imaging Archive is a collaboration of many key investigators with Fred Prior, PhD (University of Arkansas), as the principal investigator. Processes within the NCTN clinical trial groups serve to protect all information of subjects participating on clinical trials including their tissue, imaging, and radiation therapy treatment objects. Once a trial has completed accrual and primary endpoints have been recognized and published, an important objective of the National Cancer Institute is to move study information to a public archive for use by all interested in translational science and application of new informatics tools for trial analysis. The objective is for all important material including tissue biomarkers and outcome information be available to investigators. TCIA has a strong infrastructure with expertise in informatics science, imaging, digital pathology, and clinical trial management. The archive currently houses a diverse portfolio of studies and is poised to function at an enterprise level to support translational science improvement. The current portfolio of studies accessible through the TCIA includes studies involving low- and high-grade glioma with associated pathology. Over 1000 datasets are available on 11 studies. TCIA will be an invaluable resource for future translational science in neuro-oncology [20, 21]. Cancers of all disease types will be made available to investigators worldwide through this mechanism.

6. Conclusions

Neuro-oncology is an increasingly important component in the care of patients with cancer. Both primary lesions and metastatic disease affect a significant segment of the pediatric and adult populations. The care of these patients requires extended healthcare system resources for physician expertise and para health professionals for supportive and rehabilitative care. Progress will be made by optimizing uniform applications of imaging both at disease presentation and response to therapy. Informatics processes are established in the NCTN and the TCIA to help move this forward for patients afflicted with CNS disease. Information from trials will be available in a public TCIA archive to help investigators perform translational research through this mechanism and accelerate progress in this field.

Acknowledgements

U24 CA180803
U24 CA215109

Conflict of interest

The authors declare no conflict of interest.

Author details

Thomas J. FitzGerald[1*], Maryann Bishop-Jodoin[1], Fran Laurie[1], Richard Hanusik[1], Matthew Iandoli[1], Kathryn Karolczuk[1], Sandra Kessel[1], Fred Prior[2], Joel Saltz[3], Ashish Sharma[4], Michael Knopp[5], Mark Rosen[6], Ying Xiao[6], David Followill[7], Jeff Michalski[8], M. Giulia Cicchetti[1] and Janaki Moni[1]

1 University of Massachusetts/IROC Rhode Island, Lincoln, RI, USA

2 University of Arkansas/TCIA, Little Rock, AR, USA

3 Stony Brook University/TCIA, Stony Brook, NY, USA

4 Emory University/TCIA, Atlanta, GA, USA

5 Ohio State University/IROC Ohio, Columbus, OH, USA

6 University of Pennsylvania/IROC Philadelphia, Philadelphia, PA, USA

7 MD Anderson/IROC Houston, Houston, TX, USA

8 Washington University of St. Louis/IROC St. Louis, St. Louis, MO, USA

*Address all correspondence to: tjfitzgerald@qarc.org

References

[1] Glicksman AS, Reinstein LE, McShan D, Laurie F. Radiotherapy quality assurance program in a cooperative group. International Journal of Radiation Oncology, Bioliology, Physics. 1981;7:1561-1568. DOI: 10.1016/0360-3016(81)90089-4

[2] Glicksman AS, Wasserman TH, Bjarngard B, Laurie F. The structure for a radiation oncology protocol. The Committee of Radiation Oncology Group Chairmen. International Journal of Radiation Oncology, Biology, Physics. 1992;**23**:1079-1082

[3] FitzGerald TJ, Urie M, Ulin K, Laurie F, Yorty J, Hanusik R, et al. Processes for quality improvements in radiation oncology clinical trials. International Journal of Radiation Oncology, Bioliology, Physics. 2008;**71**:S76-S79. DOI: 10.1016/j.ijrobp.2007.07.2387

[4] FitzGerald TJ. What we have learned: The impact of quality from a clinical trials perspective. Seminars in Radiation Oncology. 2012;**22**:18-28. DOI: 10.1016/j.semradonc.2011.09.004

[5] FitzGerald TJ, Bishop-Jodoin M, Laurie F, O'Meara E, Davis C, Bogart J, et al. The importance of imaging in radiation oncology for National Clinical Trials Network protocols. International Journal of Radiation Oncology, Biology, Physics. 2018;**102**:775-782. DOI: 10.1016/j.ijrobp.2018.08.039

[6] Mendenhall NP, Meyer J, Williams J, et al. The impact of central quality assurance review prior to radiation therapy on protocol compliance: POG 9426, a trial in pediatric Hodgkin's disease. Blood. 2005;**106**:753. Available from: http://www.bloodjournal.org/content/106/11/753

[7] Friedman DL, Chen L, Wolden S, Buxton A, McCarten K, FitzGerald TJ, et al. Dose-intensive response-based chemotherapy and radiation therapy for children and adolescents with newly diagnosed intermediate-risk Hodgkin lymphoma: A report from the Children's oncology group study AHOD0031. Journal of Clinical Oncology. 2014;**32**:3651-3658. DOI: 10.1200/JCO.2013.52.5410

[8] Dharmarajan KV, Friedman DL, FitzGerald TJ, McCarten KM, Constine LS, Chen L, et al. Radiotherapy quality assurance report from children's oncology group AHOD0031. International Journal of Radiation Oncology, Biology, Physics. 2015;**91**:1065-1071. DOI: 10.1016/j.ijrobp.2014.11.034

[9] FitzGerald TJ, Bishop-Jodoin M, Followill D, et al. Imaging and data acquisition in clinical trials for radiation therapy. International Journal of Radiation Oncology, Biology, Physics. 2016;**94**:404-411. DOI: 10.1016/j.ijrobp 2015.10.028

[10] Ulin K, Urie MM, Cherlow JM. Results of a multi-institutional benchmark test for cranial CT/MR image registration. International Journal of Radiation Oncology, Biology, Physics. 2010;**77**:1584-1589. DOI: 10.1016/j.ijrobp.2009.10.017

[11] Gebhardt BJ, Dobelbower MC, Ennis WH, Bag AK, Markert JM, Fiveash JB. Patterns of failure for glioblastoma multiforme following limited margin radiation and concurrent Temozolomide. Radiation Oncology. 2014;**9**:130. DOI: 10.1186/1748-717X-9-130

[12] Uehara K, Sasayama T, Miyawaki D, Nishimua H, Yoshida K, Okamoto Y, et al. Patterns of failure after multimodal treatment for high-grade glioma: Effectiveness of MIB-1 labeling index. Radiation

Oncology. 2012;7:104. DOI: 10.1186/1748-717X-7-104

[13] Stall B, Zach L, Ning H, Ondos J, Arora B, Shankavaram U, et al. Comparison of T2 and FLAIR imaging for target delineation in high grade gliomas. Radiation Oncology. 2010;**5**:5. DOI: 10.1186/1748-717X-5-5

[14] Lao J, Chen Y, Li ZC, Li Q, Zhang J, Liu J, et al. A deep learning-based radiomics model for prediction of survival in glioblastoma multiforme. Scientific Reports. 2017;7:10353. DOI: 10.1038/s41598-017-10649-8

[15] Zhou M, Chaudhury B, Hall LO, Goldgof DB, Gillies RJ, Gatenby RA. Identifying spatial imaging biomarkers of glioblastoma multiforme. Journal of Magnetic Resonance Imaging. 2017;**46**:115-123. DOI: 10.1002/jmri.25497

[16] Xi YB, Guo F, Xu ZL, Li C, Wei W, Tian P, et al. Radiomics signature: A potential biomarker for the prediction of MGMT promotor methylation in glioblastoma. Journal of Magnetic Resonance Imaging. 2018;**47**:1380-1387. DOI: 10.1002/jmri.25860

[17] Eckel-Passow JE, Decker PA, Kosel ML, Kollmeyer TM, Molinaro AM, Rice T, et al. Using germline variants to estimate glioma and subtype risks. Neuro-Oncology. 2019;**21**:451-461. DOI: 10.1093/neuonc/noz009

[18] Saltz J, Sharma A, Iyer G, Bremer E, Wang F, Jasniewski A, et al. A containerized software system for generation, management, and exploration of features from whole slide tissue images. Cancer Research. 2017;77:e79-e82. DOI: 10.1158/0008-5472.CAN-17-0316

[19] Cooper LA, Kong J, Gutman DA, Wang F, Gao J, Appin C, et al. Integrated morphologic analysis for the identification and characterization of disease subtypes. Journal of the American Medical Informatics Association. 2012;**19**:317-323. DOI: 10.1136/amiajnl-2011-000700

[20] Prior F, Smith K, Sharma A, Kirby J, Tarbox L, Clark K, et al. The public cancer radiology imaging collections of the cancer imaging archive. Scientific Data. 2017;**4**:170124. DOI: 10.1038/sdata.2017.124

[21] Prior F, Almeida J, Kathiravelu P, Kurc T, Smith K, Fitzgerald TJ, et al. Open access image repositories: High quality data to enable machine learning research. Clinical Radiology. 2019. pii: S0009-9260(19)30169-2. DOI: 10.1016/j.crad.2019.04.002 [Epub ahead of print]